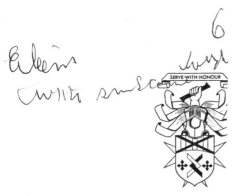

Fight Old Age

with

THE WALKER-NADDELL
TRAINING PROGRAMME

by

ALEXANDER WALKER-NADDELL
FRCS, FRCPS, FSA (Scot.), FRSA, K.St.J, ERD, JP, DL
Consultant Orthopaedic and Neuro Surgeon

Edited by —
ANNIE E. LIVESEY, MA

Published by —
J. R. REID PRINTERS LTD., BLANTYRE, GLASGOW

Typeset in 10 point English Times
on Compugraphic MCS8400 Phototypesetter

© Alexander Walker-Naddell 1987

ISBN 0 948785 01 2

Typeset, Printed and Published in Scotland by
J. R. Reid Printers Ltd., Blantyre, Glasgow.

Foreword

WALKER-NADDELL is a man possessed of a lively mind, dogged determination and an independent spirit: qualities which have enabled doctors and scientists throughout the ages to extend the boundaries of existing knowledge.

Although he is thoroughly trained and experienced in traditional medicine, he has never been afraid to question current conventional treatments and, if necessary, to find alternative and better solutions to the problems in hand. Such techniques seldom evolve easily or quickly. The original inspiration must be supported and developed by years of study and experiment. It requires a tenacity of purpose, much courage and an inner confidence to continue along one's line of research sometimes in the face of criticism by colleagues.

The story of Walker-Naddell's discovery of a unique treatment to cure the slipped disc condition has already been told in a previous book, 'The Slipped Disc and the Aching Back of Man'. Such were his convictions about this technique that he set up in private practice to prove and develop this new treatment. He has now completed much original research into the condition of migraine and its causes — a story still to be told.

In this book, however, he discusses a completely different and unusual approach to the ageing process. He maintains that most of, if not all the physical changes that seem to come inevitably with old age can be prevented. He rejects the idea of a passive acceptance of the constraints that commonly develop in old age. By exercising sensibly and regularly according to a programme he has devised he insists that we can remain active and virtually painfree right into very old age. He invites us all, young and old, to accept the challenge of Old Age and fight it daily with the Walker-Naddell Training Programme.

NAN LIVESEY
Editor

To my children:
Gail, Victoria and John

Acknowledgements

THIS book in many ways complements my earlier one, 'The Slipped Disc and the Aching Back of Man' that deals, in particular, with the slipped disc condition but also with many other back problems. Many of my patients are elderly and in the course of treating them I have become increasingly interested in the ageing process in general. My research into this has spanned over many years and for some time I have wanted to collate my results and ideas on the subject in book form.

Its realisation has been achieved with the loyal support of friends and colleagues. Especially, I should like to express my most grateful thanks to my editor, Nan Livesey whose assiduous care was invaluable in helping to formulate the book and secondly, to John Reid, my printer and publisher, whose highly professional skills eased the task of finally getting the book into print.

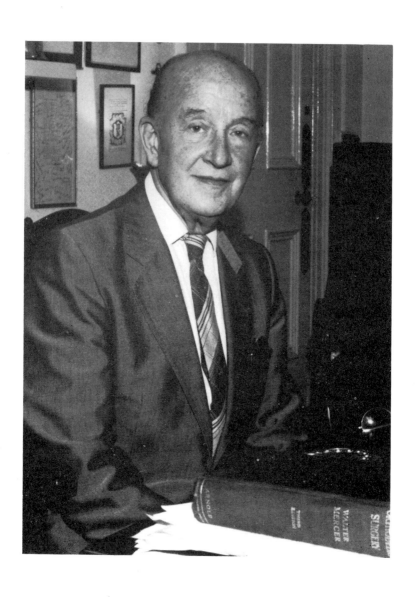

The Author

Fight Old Age
with the
Walker-Naddell Training Programme

WHY GROW OLD?

KEEP fit, keep healthy and stay looking young!

In this book I hope to demonstrate that exercise will keep you not only looking fitter and younger, but more importantly keep at bay many of the adverse effects of ageing. Old age in the terms of the years we live cannot be denied but I believe that **we need not** accept many of the changes that seem to develop naturally with advancing years. That one should relax and grow old gracefully is **not** a good maxim. There are many ways, I believe, to combat the process of old age and remain healthier, vital and more active right into very old age.

Good posture, a supple body and a spring in the step are the hallmarks of good health and youthful vitality. A good carriage not only provides the basis for an attractive well-dressed appearance but also for one of health, strength and youth.

One of the first signs of **ageing,** or even debility caused by illness, is walking with the head bent forwards and a slight rounding of the shoulders. The reason for this is quite obvious if one considers that in most everyday activities, including eating, drinking, even sleeping, the head is held slightly bent forwards for long periods. For complete relaxation people usually adopt a position of forward flexion of the whole body slumping forwards with a curved spine and dropped head in their arm chairs. Even before birth whilst still in the womb the foetus adopts a similar position: the head and spinal column in a complete state of forward flexion. Rarely does anyone extend the head backwards to look at the sky. Seldom does a person spend more than 10 seconds in a 24 hour period with the head bent backwards. Thus the muscles at the back of the neck are most vulnerable to strain and possible overstretching. This very often results in faulty posture leading to the development of a 'Dowager's Hump' at the base of the neck. This is the first stage and indeed the prime cause of further deformities which we all associate with the ageing process. Such habitual bad posture leads to further strain to form a 'Humpback'. This rounding may extend downwards to become a complete 'Round Back', involving the lower or lumbar area of the spinal column. If this is not corrected the spinal column becomes fixed and painful and the person concerned will be unable to stand and walk erect.

The other significant cause of problems in old age is the onset òf arthritis which affects most people of 40 or over and causes stiffness, thickening, swelling and possible pain in the joints. This condition is exaggerated by faulty alignment of the joints, which is a direct result of the extra pressure on these joints caused by defective posture.

In order to combat both these factors that so greatly contribute to the ageing process my training programme will exercise the muscles at the back of the neck, in particular, and those that support the spinal column throughout its length and also it will keep the joints most subject to arthritis, mobile and painfree ensuring both good posture and a youthful freedom of movement.

Various courses of exercises are readily available now both in print and on tape, so why another? and why is mine, the Walker-Naddell training programme so special? There are many important reasons.

1. I used my experience as a qualified doctor and surgeon to formulate the programme and thus it carries with it the seal of medical approval!

2. It was devised not only as a keep-fit programme but also to prevent or combat all outward signs of ageing: in particular, to maintain good posture and supple joints.

3. The exercises can be done by young or old, at whatever stage of fitness they may be. They are suitable for all, because they were designed as part of the treatment for correcting the deformities that may come with old age if they are allowed to develop (see Part Two). They are definitely not injurious to health!

4. They can be done anywhere, at any time, for they require no apparatus.

5. They take no more than three or four minutes per training session and thus can be fitted into even the tightest business schedule. It is recommended that the exercises are done each morning and evening. Thus the total time spent will be less than 10 minutes each day.

6. They form a complete and systematic programme designed to exercise in turn every single muscle, especially those that support the head and back and to keep the joints most subject to arthritis, mobile and painfree. Deep breaths should be taken whilst exercising to provide oxygen necessary for muscle regeneration.

That exercise helps to keep the body fit and healthy is now widely accepted. However, as people go into middle age, there is a tendency, possibly because of business and family commitments, to take less and less exercise. Yet it is often at this time that heart conditions may occur and arthritis develop — the very time indeed that people require to exercise systematically, but **carefully,** to prevent the onset of old age.

This tendency to become less active leads to general lack of muscle movement and thus of muscle tone. Thus weakness of muscles will occur in areas of greatest stress. The weight of the head puts considerable and constant strain on the neck muscles, especially those at the back (or posterior) of the neck. As we have explained in nearly all everyday activities the head is bent forwards: in eating, writing, drawing, gardening and even in sleep. Many occupations exaggerate this stress for they demand the head be held forward for prolonged periods. Eventually the posterior muscles of the neck may become overstretched and thus produce the first outward sign of ageing. Even as early as late middle age people tend to walk with the head bent forward and the shoulders slightly rounded.

Most people accept the fact that by the time they reach the age of 70, or even younger, the ageing process will leave them with a permanent stoop or bowing of the back. This posture leads to further deformities, for the older person may now feel he will fall forwards as he walks. He unconsciously seeks to restore his balance by bending the knees forwards. This, not only impairs mobility but also puts excess pressure on the hip and knee joints and eventually also on to the ankle joints. They may become swollen and painful and thus impede normal walking. The weight of the whole trunk is now transferred to the feet which causes them to lose their natural spring and the arches of the foot to flatten. The gait of the elderly person is now grossly affected and he is obliged to adopt a shuffling gait in order to remain restrictedly mobile. With such restricted mobility, the joints of the body become more inflexible and the muscles waste or atrophy through disuse.

Most people regard these changes as inevitable, for they can occur in the normal healthy ageing person. However, I believe that if my Training Programme is carried out regularly, none of this is necessary, though it is true that, by accepting the first signs of ageing, the other deformities may gradually follow.

Exercise, like most other things is subject to fashion and I question the current vogue for **jogging.** It may well have stimulated those not interested in other types of sport — or for whom these are not readily available — to get out of their armchairs in front of the television and take some exercise. For the older age groups, however, it may not be ideal. The physical stress of jogging if the individual is over 40 years of age and carrying some excess weight, puts a strain on the vital organs of the jogger. He, or she may, for example, be suffering from early features of cardio-vascular disease or the onset of arthritis in the foot, ankle, knee and/or hip joints. In these conditions jogging may result in more harm than good.

Swimming, on the other hand is an excellent exercise, especially breast stroke. Muscles are brought into action and kept in tone and the depth of breathing required for swimming provides oxygen which tones the whole muscular system. The buoyancy of the water prevents weight being exerted on to the body and avoids stress and strains on the joints. Some people unfortunately have never learnt how to swim but it is **never** too late to start. They would find it rewarding of itself as well as beneficial for their physical being. In addition, it is a sport that can usually be carried on right into very old age.

Sport, of any kind, provides not only exercise but good companionship, competitiveness and a welcome break from the routine of office or home. However, it is not necessarily enough, for each type of sport may only exercise certain areas of the body and, in any case, time and opportunity for such activities may be restricted. Following a systematic training programme ensures that **all** the muscles and joints of the body are being kept in tone and sportsmen will usually find their game will benefit from this routine of exercises.

The first section of this book sets out the complete training programme in order, starting with the exercises that tone the muscles of the three areas of the back: the neck or cervical, the upper back or dorsal, the lower back or lumbar. Next follow the exercises designed to combat the onset of arthritis in specific joints, taken in order: the shoulder, the elbow, the wrists and finger joints, the hip, ankle, and the joints of the feet. The second section of the book describes the deformities that often do occur in old age and the exercises where appropriate are repeated as part of the treatment suggested.

It is, however, much more important to start exercising the whole body **before** the deformity begins to arise. The awareness of the weaknesses that may come with age will, I hope, encourage people to adopt the training programme as a form of **preventative medicine** that requires far less effort **NOW** than later and, in the long run, will prevent pain and restricted mobility as they get older. These programmes are suitable for any age of patient and form a good basic exercise routine at whatever the level of fitness of the subject. Younger age groups will usually play various types of sport in addition and these exercises will improve their play. It is recommended that everyone should acquire the habit of twice daily exercises as part of their normal day, so that it becomes as routine as washing or the cleaning of teeth.

PART ONE

THE WALKER-NADDELL TRAINING PROGRAMME

Before starting the training programme it is important to remember:

1. The exercises should be done regularly and this comes more easily if a **daily routine** is observed: preferably doing them night and morning.

2. Deep breaths must be taken throughout. Regular deep breathing prevents overtiring of the muscles and without oxygen muscles out of tone will not easily regenerate. Without deep breathing there is a retention of carbon dioxide and lactic acid in the muscles being exercised.

3. When performing exercises in the erect posture make sure that some degree of stability is achieved. For extra stability stand with legs a foot apart instead of close together. Older people may prefer to sit to do the exercises wherever possible.

4. When a chair is required make sure that it is strong and well balanced so that weight exerted on its back will not cause it to fall over.

5. In all exercises all muscles being moved should be kept taut to permit maximum movement in all joints.

THE WALKER-NADDELL TRAINING PROGRAMME FOR NECK OR CERVICAL AREA

Exercise I

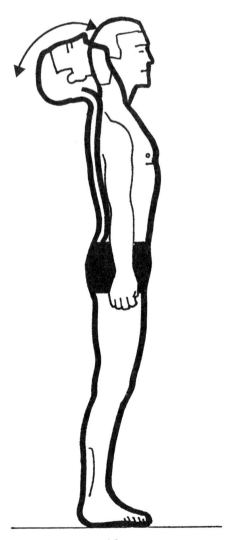

THE COMPLETE WALKER-NADDELL
TRAINING PROGRAMME

THE NECK OR CERVICAL AREA

Exercise I

1. Stand erect with feet slightly apart. Older people may prefer to sit for Exercises I and II.

2. Jerk the head backwards, and then forwards but only as far as the erect posture, (never bending the neck forwards).

3. Repeat five times.

THE WALKER-NADDELL TRAINING PROGRAMME FOR NECK OR CERVICAL AREA

Exercise II

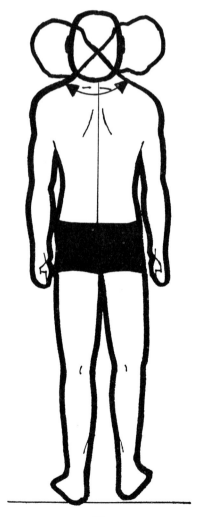

NECK OR CERVICAL AREA

Exercise II

1. Stand erect with feet slightly apart.

2. Hold the head backwards.

3. Rotate the head in this axis, ear to shoulder, five times to one side and five times to the opposite side. Avoid bringing the head forwards beyond the shoulder point.

4. The rotation should follow the course of the round part of a capital 'D'. The head should never be rotated round and round as this will cause dizziness.

THE WALKER-NADDELL TRAINING PROGRAMME FOR NECK OR CERVICAL AREA

Exercise III

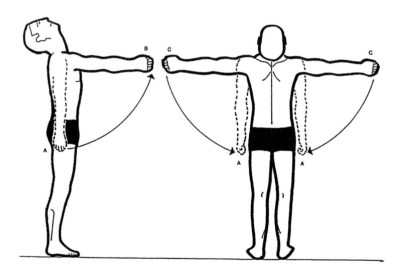

NECK OR CERVICAL AREA

Exercise III

1. Stand erect with feet slightly apart.

2. Hold the head back, looking up to the ceiling.

3. Stretch the arms out straight in front and parallel to the floor.

4. With the elbow joints fixed and fists clenched rotate the stiff arms quickly backwards as if swimming breast stroke, with the shoulder blades coming together when the arms are tight back.

5. Swing the stiff arms down past the body and repeat five times. Take a deep breath when the arms are being raised to the horizontal plane, and exhale as the shoulder blades are brought together.

THE WALKER-NADDELL TRAINING PROGRAMME FOR NECK OR CERVICAL AREA

Exercise IV

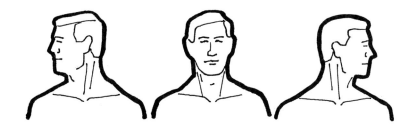

NECK OR CERVICAL AREA

Exercise IV

1. The patient may sit or stand for this exercise.

2. With the head erect and looking forward, turn the neck slowly but firmly sideways, until the chin is in line with the top of the shoulder. Then pause for a count of five.

3. Perform the exercise five times in each direction.

THE WALKER-NADDELL TRAINING PROGRAMME FOR UPPER BACK OR DORSAL AREA

Exercise I

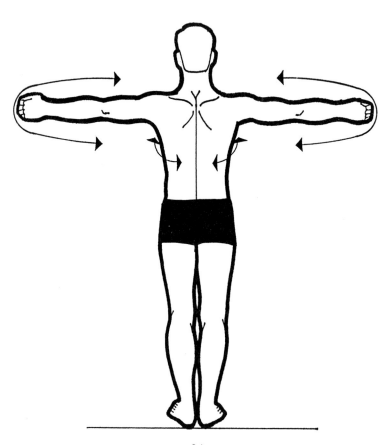

THE UPPER BACK OR DORSAL AREA

Exercise I

1. Stand in the erect posture, with feet together, or slightly apart for extra stability.

2. With stiff elbow and wrist joints and clenched fists stretch the arms out sideways at shoulder level, parallel to the floor.

3. Holding this posture, whip the arms first one way and then the other, rotating the chest as far as it will go, from side to side. This, in turn, rotates the dorsal or thoracic vertebrae.

4. Repeat five times in each direction.

5. Breathe in and out with each movement.

THE WALKER-NADDELL TRAINING PROGRAMME FOR UPPER BACK OR DORSAL AREA

Excercise II

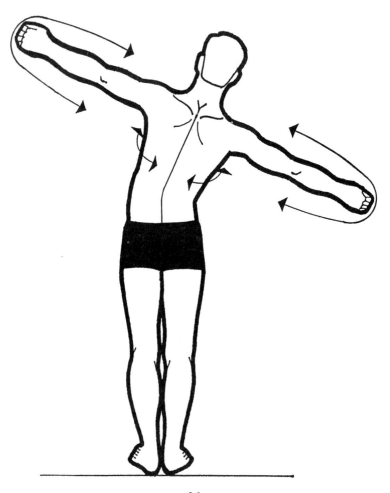

UPPER BACK OR DORSAL AREA

Exercise II

1. Stand in the erect posture with feet together, or slightly apart for extra stability.

2. With stiff elbows and wrist joints and clenched fists stretch the arms out sideways at shoulder level, parallel to the floor.

3. Lower one arm, bending at the waist with the other pointing upwards, still with the arm straight and in line with the tip of the shoulders.

4. Holding this posture, whip the arms first one way and then the other.

5. Repeat five times in each direction.

6. Repeat five further times with the chest flexed at the waist in the opposite direction.

7. Inhale and exhale regularly to prevent overtiring of the muscles.

THE WALKER-NADDELL TRAINING PROGRAMME FOR UPPER BACK OR DORSAL AREA

Exercise III

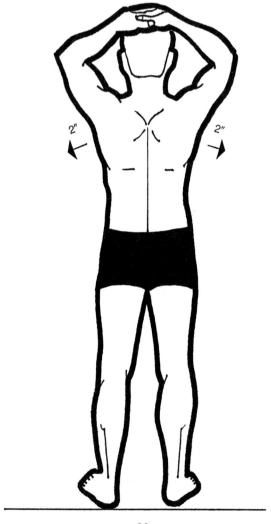

UPPER BACK OR DORSAL AREA

Exercise III

1. The patient may either sit or stand.

2. Clasp hands on the top of the head, with elbows raised as high as possible.

3. Swing the chest from side to side for about 2″, extending upwards with every movement.

4. Repeat five times in each direction.

THE WALKER-NADDELL TRAINING PROGRAMME FOR UPPER BACK OR DORSAL AREA

Exercise IV

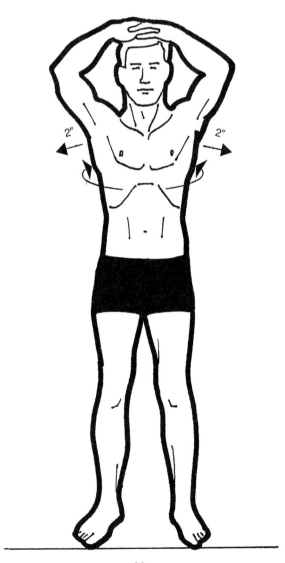

UPPER BACK OR DORSAL AREA

Exercise IV

1. Adopt the same posture as for Exercise III.
2. Rotate the chest, bending 2″ in all directions.
3. Repeat five times one way and five times the other.

THE WALKER-NADDELL TRAINING PROGRAMME FOR LOWER BACK OR LUMBAR AREA

Exercise I

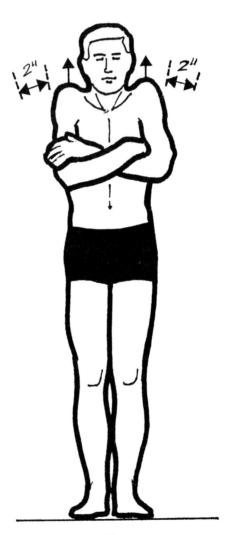

LOWER BACK OR LUMBAR AREA

Exercise I

MUSCLE TONING TRACTION

1. Stand erect with feet together, or slightly apart for extra stability.

2. Expand the chest. This increases lumbar curve.

3. Fold arms across chest.

4. Raise points of shoulders to ears.

5. In this posture move the chest for 2″ from side to side 10 times each way, bending through waist.

6. Take a deep breath with each movement. The shoulders should remain fixed in this position. It is the chest which moves from side to side and at the same time it is being gradually pulled upwards.

THE WALKER-NADDELL TRAINING PROGRAMME FOR LOWER BACK OR LUMBAR AREA

Exercise II

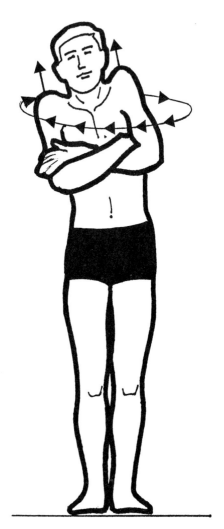

LOWER BACK OR LUMBAR AREA

Exercise II

MUSCLE TONING TRACTION WITH SPINAL ROTATION

1. Adopt the same posture as in Exercise I.

2. Rotate the chest through the waistline round and round for no more than 2″ from the vertical — first five times in one direction and then five times in the other direction.

THE WALKER-NADDELL TRAINING PROGRAMME FOR LOWER BACK OR LUMBAR AREA

Exercise III

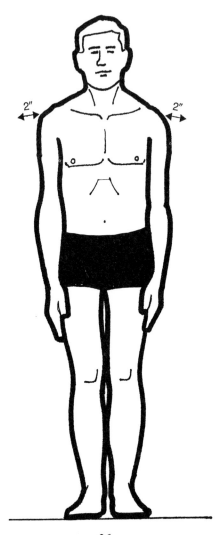

LOWER BACK OR LUMBAR AREA

Exercise III

PENDULUM MOVEMENT OF THE TRUNK

1. Stand in the erect posture with the arms kept at the side of the body.

2. Keep the chest expanded to increase the lumbar curve or lordosis.

3. Flex the chest laterally 10 times from side to side 2″ in either direction at speed. Bend at the waist only. Do not move legs. The shoulders are held fixed and only move with the chest.

THE WALKER-NADDELL TRAINING PROGRAMME FOR LOWER BACK OR LUMBAR AREA

Exercise IV

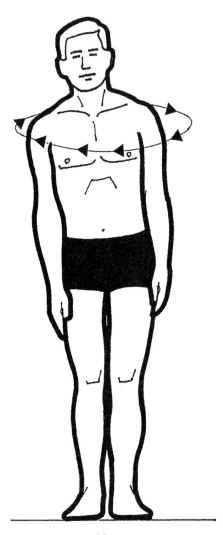

LOWER BACK OR LUMBAR AREA

Exercise IV

ROTATION OF THE TRUNK THROUGH THE WAIST LINE

1. Stand in the erect posture as in Exercise III.

2. Rotate the chest, bending at waist line only, not more than 2″, five times in one direction and five times in the other.

3. Arms are kept close to body.

4. Shoulders are not raised, but move with the chest.

THE WALKER-NADDELL TRAINING PROGRAMME FOR SHOULDER JOINTS

Exercise I

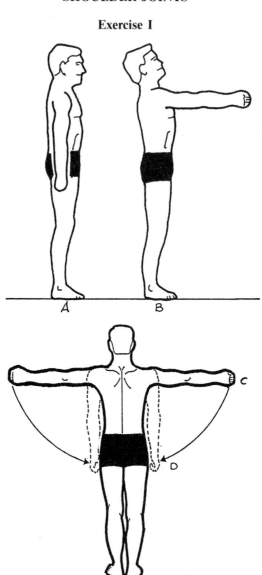

SHOULDER JOINTS

Exercise I

1. Stand erect, with feet slightly apart.

2. With clenched fists and straight taut arms, raise the arms from the side of the body forwards and upwards to shoulder level — unless pain is experienced. In this case raise the arms to a position **always** just **short** of pain.

3. From this position (and it may not be at shoulder level) move the arms round in a breast stroke movement, round and back to the sides of the body.

4. This should be done five times.

5. Eventually the pain and stiffness (if any) will disappear and the exercise should then (and only then) be done at shoulder level.

THE WALKER-NADDELL TRAINING PROGRAMME FOR SHOULDER JOINTS

Exercise II

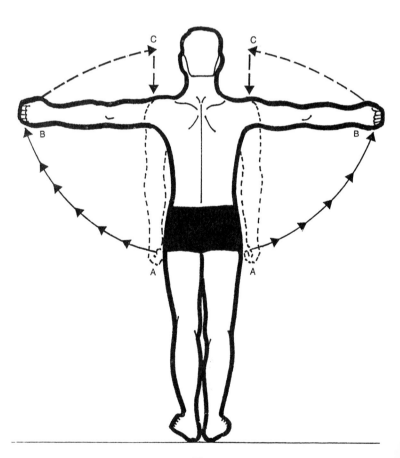

SHOULDER JOINTS

Exercise II

Reverse the rotation of Exercise I, holding the same position arms raised to shoulder level, first moving the arms backwards and then rotating forwards until the hands are to the side of the body again. This should be done five times.

If pain is experienced the exercise should be performed at a level without pain.

Day by day and very gradually, the patient will notice that the level, to which he can lift his arms without pain to begin the exercise will be raised. The exercise should then be done at shoulder level.

THE WALKER-NADDELL TRAINING PROGRAMME FOR SHOULDER JOINTS

Exercise III

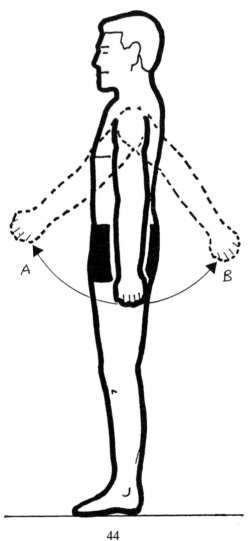

SHOULDER JOINTS

Exercise III

1. Adopt the same position as in I and II with clenched fists and arms like rods.

2. Swing the arms parallel to the sides of the body forwards and backwards, slowly as far as possible **without** pain. Avoid any jerky movement.

3. This should be done five times.

THE WALKER-NADDELL TRAINING PROGRAMME FOR SHOULDER JOINTS

Exercise IV

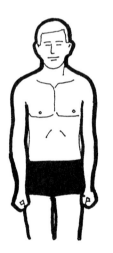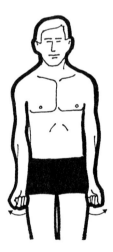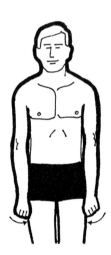

SHOULDER JOINTS

Exercise IV

1. Adopt the same position as in I, II and III with the fists clenched and the arms taut like rods.

2. Hold the arms close to the sides of the body and rotate the upper arms, one way and then the other, using a screwdriver type of action, as if 'driving' a screw into the ground.

3. This should be done five times.

THE WALKER-NADDELL TRAINING PROGRAMME FOR ELBOW JOINTS

Exercise I

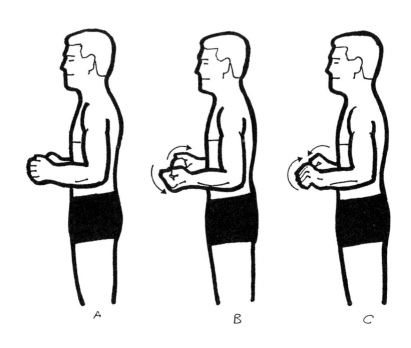

A   B   C

ELBOW JOINTS

Exercise I

1. The patient may sit or stand but the latter is perhaps preferable.

2. The arms should be bent at the elbows to form a right angle.

3. The fists should be clenched at all times and the wrists kept straight with the forearms.

4. Holding the upper arms firmly into the side of the body the forearms should be rotated through the elbow joints slowly and firmly, first one way and then the other, five times.

THE WALKER-NADDELL TRAINING PROGRAMME FOR WRIST JOINTS

Exercise I

Rotation

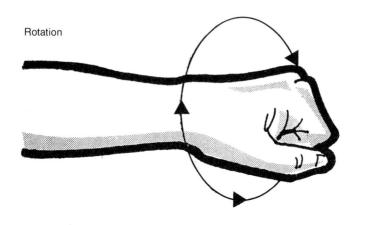

A

Rotation in reverse

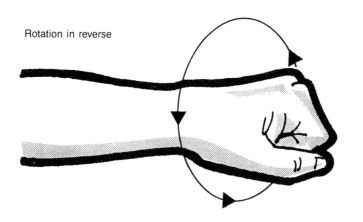

B

WRIST JOINTS

Exercise I

1. The exercise may be done sitting or standing.

2. Bend the arms at the elbow and keep the arm taut, with fists clenched. Hold the arms into the side of the body.

3. Rotate hands through the wrist joints, five times in one direction and five times in the opposite direction.

THE WALKER-NADDELL TRAINING PROGRAMME FOR WRIST JOINTS

Exercise II

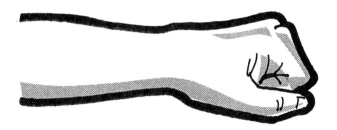

A

Dorsi flexion

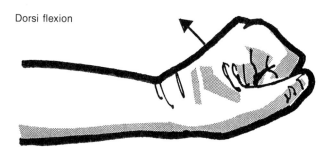

B

Palmar flexion

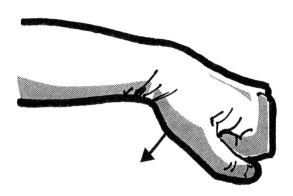

C

WRIST JOINTS

Exercise II

1. Adopt the same position as for Exercise I.

2. With fists clenched bend the hands up and down from the wrists. Ten movements in all, five up and five down.

FINGER JOINTS

Stiffening of the finger joints is very common in the elderly and thus dexterity may be grossly impeded. To prevent this, older people should exercise the fingers in the following way.

Exercise I

Flex the fingers up and down in sequence, as if playing scales on a piano.

Exercise II

Stretch the hand in order to separate the fingers as far as possible and hold the hand in this position for a minute, or say, for a count of 20.

THE WALKER-NADDELL TRAINING PROGRAMME FOR HIP JOINTS

Exercise I

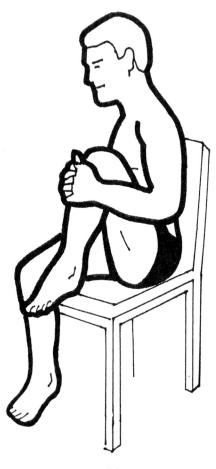

HIP JOINTS

Exercise I

1. Sit on a strong dining chair.
2. With hands clasped in front of the knee joint pull the leg up to the chest wall and hold for a count of five.
3. Repeat for the other limb.

HIP JOINTS

Exercise II

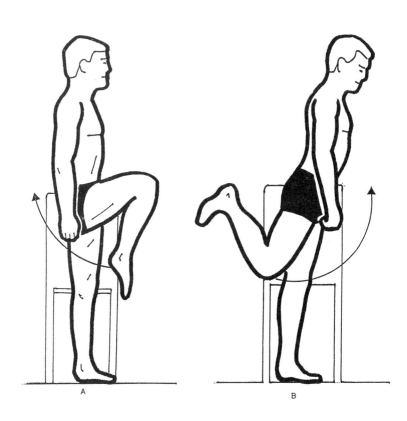

Forward Flexion of the Hip Joint
with Backward Extension.

HIP JOINTS

Exercise II

1. Stand with left hand holding the back of a strong dining chair.

2. Bend the right knee at right angles to the thigh and hold this position throughout.

3. Bump with vigour upwards and backwards (the knee still bent at right angles to thigh) five times.

4. Exercise the left limb, similarly.

THE WALKER-NADDELL TRAINING PROGRAMME FOR HIP JOINTS

Exercise III

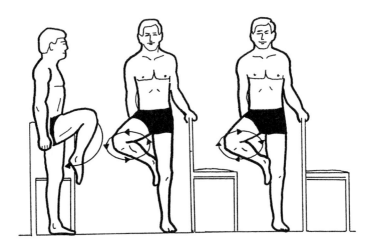

HIP JOINTS

Exercise III

1. Stand, holding the back of a strong dining chair with the left hand.

2. Raise the right knee upwards as high as is comfortable keeping the knee bent. Rotate the knee outwards, to follow a circular movement, back past the other knee. Repeat this five times, and five rotating inwards. Similarly exercise the left limb by changing positions and holding the back of the chair with the right hand.

THE WALKER-NADDELL TRAINING PROGRAMME FOR KNEE JOINTS

Exercise I

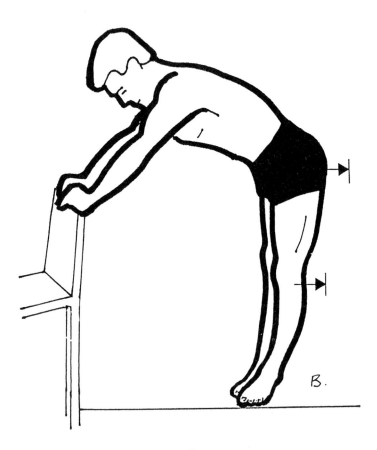

KNEE JOINTS

Exercise I

1. Stand behind a strong high-backed chair about a foot away from it.

2. Rest the hands on the back of the chair.

3. Rise up on the toes and pull the knee joints backwards as far as possible.

4. Bend the trunk towards the top of the chair, without touching it, still ensuring the knee joints are pulled backwards. Hold in this position initially for a count of five.

THE WALKER-NADDELL TRAINING PROGRAMME FOR KNEE JOINTS

Exercise II

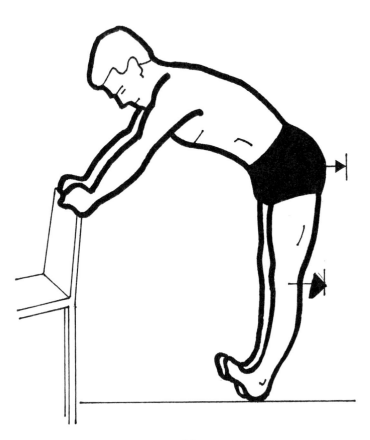

KNEE JOINTS

Exercise II

1. Adopt the same attitude as for Exercise I, again resting the hands on the back of the chair and standing about a foot behind it.

2. Rise up on the heels, with toes pointing towards the chin.

3. Pull the knee joints backwards as far as possible despite the pain involved.

4. Bend the chest towards the top of the chair without touching it, still pulling the knee joints backwards regardless of pain and hold for a count of five.

THE WALKER-NADDELL TRAINING PROGRAMME FOR ANKLE JOINTS

Exercise I

Dorsi Flexion of the Ankle Joint.

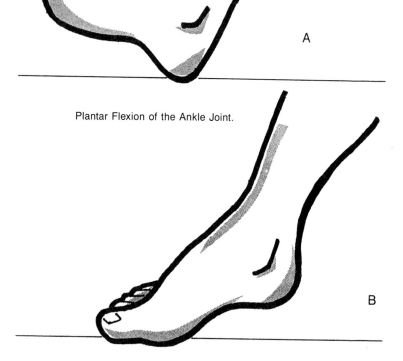

A

Plantar Flexion of the Ankle Joint.

B

Extension and Flexion of the Ankle Joint.

ANKLE JOINTS

Exercise I

Exercises I and II should be carried out sitting down.

The ankle joint is flexed up and down five times exercising each foot in turn.

Ensure that all the toes are curled downwards as far as possible towards the sole of the foot in this and the following exercise. This helps to keep the muscles of the arch of the foot just below the toes in good tone.

THE WALKER-NADDELL TRAINING PROGRAMME FOR ANKLE JOINTS

Exercise II

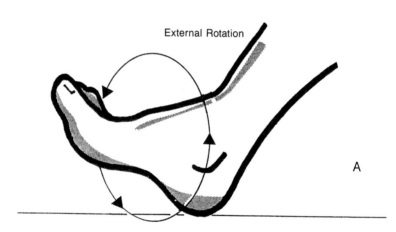

External Rotation

A

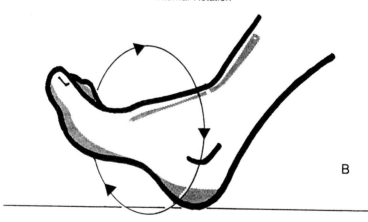

Internal Rotation

B

Rotation of the Ankle Joint.

68

ANKLE JOINTS

Exercise II

Rotate the ankle joint, first inwardly five times and then in the opposite direction five times, exercising each foot in turn.

These movements prevent the formation of bony adhesions, contraction of the ligaments and gradually they will tone up the muscles which control the ankle joint movements.

THE WALKER-NADDELL TRAINING PROGRAMME FOR ANKLE JOINTS

Exercise III

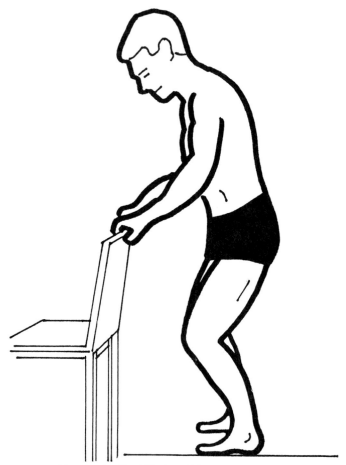

Exercise for Dorsi Flexion of the Ankle Joints.

70

ANKLE JOINTS

Exercise III

1. Stand behind a strong dining chair and hold the back with both hands.

2. Feet should be about a foot behind the chair, flat on the ground.

3. Bend the knees forwards as far as possible with the feet still remaining flat on the floor.

4. Hold in this position for a count of 10, later 20.

THE WALKER-NADDELL TRAINING PROGRAMME FOR JOINTS OF THE FEET

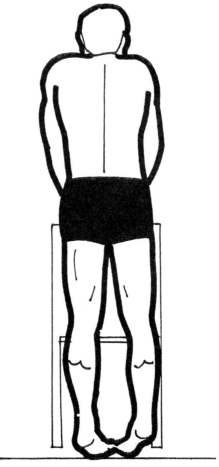

Exercise for Flat Feet.

JOINTS OF THE FEET

Exercises to tone the arches of the feet

ANTERIOR ARCH

The exercises for the ankle joint will also tone the muscles of this arch if the toes are curled downwards.

LONGITUDINAL ARCH

Exercise I

1. Stand behind a high backed chair, about a foot behind it and hold the back of the chair with both hands.

2. Rise onto toes as high as possible, with feet together.

3. In this position separate both heels as far as possible, keeping great toes together.

4. Hold this position for a count of 20.

PART TWO

The Description and Treatment
of the Deformities
of the Aged

THE AGEING PROCESS

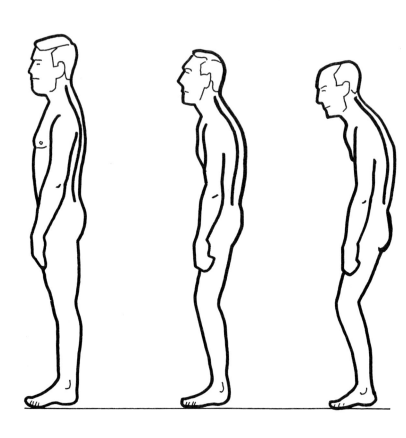

THE AGEING PROCESS

Fig. I   Normal Contour
Note that the alignment of the vertebrae, one to the other, gives rise to the specific shape of the spinal column, but this shape is maintained entirely by the muscles that surround the column.

Fig. II   The Ageing Man
Note: The slight forward flexion of the head
the slight rounding of the back
the flattening of the anterior chest wall
the slight forward flexion of the knee joints
the tendency towards flat feet, with a loss of spring in walking

In this posture the patient's activities become grossly diminished. Thus stiffening of all joints follows with a varying degree of muscle wasting. The individual's balance may become seriously impaired.

Fig. III   The Aged Man
Note: The ageing processes, referred to in the notes of Fig. II above, become exaggerated, resulting in the contraction of joint capsules and muscle wasting; the stiffening and loss of movements in most of the joints and, of course, considerable loss of height, say 7″ or more. The patient's balance is impaired, giving him a tendency to fall forward. The erect posture is maintained by the compensatory action of bending the knees forward. The consequent reduction of mobility, in especially the joints of the lower limbs, may result in a shuffling gait.

CHAPTER ONE

The Causes and Development of the Deformities of the Aged

THE normal contour of the spinal column is formed initially by the articulation of the vertebrae, one with the other, throughout the whole column. At the upper end the first cervical vertebra articulates with the condyles, or base of the skull, and at the lower aspect the fifth lumbar vertebra articulates with the upper surface of the sacrum. The specific alignment of the column is thus formed by the articulation of these joints but this normal contour is entirely controlled and maintained by the muscles that surround and control the column. Thus any weakness of this musculature may cause deformities to arise in the column.

As one gets older, one tends to become less and less active. This leads to a **disuse atrophy of the muscular system** which, in turn, diminishes joint movement, with the inevitable contraction of the joint capsules. Thus varying degrees of joint stiffness will ensue, often causing pain. The pain will again limit movement and the condition will accelerate, varying naturally from person to person. The patient will gradually become thinner with a marked loss of tone in the muscle groups, which normally move the affected joint or joints.

With the loss of muscle tone, especially in the posterior cervical, dorsal and lumbar areas of the back, **postural deformities** frequently develop in the older person. These are very often exaggerated by the type of work in which the person is engaged. Constant bending of, for e.g. the neck, as in writing or of the back as in gardening may cause the muscles supporting the head or back to become overstretched and if the person is unaware of this happening, these conditions may eventually lead to a 'Dowager's Hump' and/or 'Round Back' (see page 84). These, in turn, lead to further deformities of the lower limbs, a marked disruption of the normal gait and eventually increased reduction in mobility. These are described in detail in the next chapter.

Most elderly people are subject to **arthritis** which leads to pain and stiffness in the affected joints and may cause some deformity and a lack of mobility. There are, however, different types of arthritis

79

and some distinction should be made between the two major types. Both come under the heading of Arthritis Deformans.

ARTHRITIS DEFORMANS

Arthritis is an inflammation of the joint and **deformans** is the deformity that occurs as a result of this condition. Arthritis is a chronic inflammatory infection of the joints, (the cause of which in the majority of cases is not known), with involvement of the synovial membranes (or joint capsules), the periarticular tissues of the cartilage and the bones of the affected joint.

The condition may affect all age groups from the youngest child to the very old. The clinical picture has been written up with a specific tendency to classify according to age. This is the correct way to assess cases but it should be kept in mind that it can occur, regardless of age.

The two main types of arthritis are **Rheumatoid Arthritis** and **Osteoarthritis** but, in between, are intermediate forms and it is not certain whether these are separate entities or manifestations of the same disease in different age groups.

RHEUMATOID ARTHRITIS occurs in early adult life usually between 20-40 years of age. It is a periarticular type of arthritis, in which the painful swelling is followed by marked contractures and deformity in and around the affected joints.

OSTEOARTHRITIS usually occurs from the age of 40 to 60 years. There is usually little swelling but marked changes take place in the cartilage and bones. A monoarticular type also occurs affecting chiefly the hip, knee or shoulder joints. This type usually occurs from the age of 35 into old age. Thus it is osteoarthritis that most commonly affects the elderly and with which we are most concerned here. However, patients of whatever age, suffering deformities from other types of arthritis that may have been sustained when they were young, can be treated in exactly the same manner as the elderly with similar deformities that have resulted from osteoarthritis. Osteoarthritis causes pain with stiffness in the joints and results in lack of mobility in the patient, and consequential muscle dystrophy or wasting.

In an affected joint the process first attacks the soft structure around the joint and, later, spreads to the cartilage and bone. The synovial membrane, or capsule of the joint, becomes thickened. The cartilage cells multiply and the peripheral cells burst into the joint. If the numbers are great the joint fluid becomes turbid and the cartilage of the joint surfaces becomes roughened. This leads to lipping and osteophytic outgrowths may be formed as some cartilage cells subsequently ossify. The unossified cartilage cells tend to soften and are worn away on pressure-bearing surfaces with resulting erosion. The underlying bone when exposed reacts to eburnation of the opposing joint surfaces.

This is an important fact in the treatment of opposing arthritic joint surfaces. I use it at all times when treating arthritis. By simply rubbing one rough surface against the other the rough surfaces become smooth and polished. It can be compared to rubbing two pieces of sandpaper together. The roughness or 'spikes' of the sandpaper are worn down and become smooth. Similarly the joint surfaces become polished and smooth or eburnated.

DECALCIFICATION is also a common factor in the ageing process. It is commonly associated with osteoporosis (see appendix) which, in turn, leads to deformity in most cases. A course of calcium with Vitamin D and the use of a training programme often produces quite dramatic results. I prescribe a tablet of five mg. of calcium with Vitamin D added, to be taken in the middle of each meal, in order to allow for the absorption of the calcium and Vitamin D during the digestive process. The addition of the Vitamin D is important, for without it, calcium will not be absorbed. The practice of the exercises of the training programme will encourage mobility of the joints and also smooth the opposing surfaces of the joints i.e. eburnation of the joint surfaces to reduce pain during movement. The exercises will tone up the muscles supporting the spinal column, the upper and lower limbs and thus start correcting any previous deformity.

Thus any or all of these factors:

1. muscular weakness or dystrophy
2. habitually bad posture
3. the effects of osteoarthritis
4. the effects of decalcification of bone with osteoporosis,

all these may cause deformities to arise affecting part of or the whole skeletal system of the body, in particular the weight-bearing joints.

81

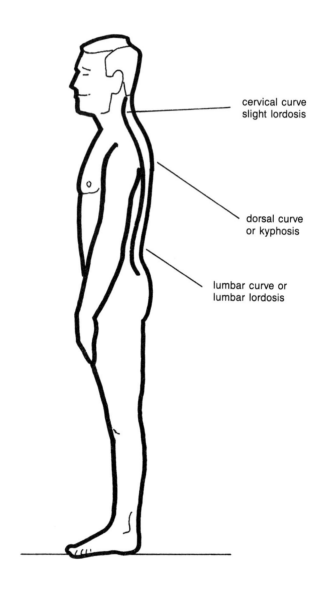

cervical curve
slight lordosis

dorsal curve
or kyphosis

lumbar curve or
lumbar lordosis

Normal Adult Contour of a Spinal Column in the Erect Posture.

CHAPTER TWO

The Deformities of the Aged

IT IS the normally accepted practice that during the examination of a patient, the doctor or consultant always works from his knowledge of the healthy body, in order to recognise the malfunction or deformity in the system. Thus in the context of this book the doctor must be able to recognise the normal contour of the spinal column to be able to assess the slightest mal-alignment.

THE NORMAL CONTOUR

When an adult stands erect the balance of the trunk is preserved by concavity alternating with convexity. Curvature of the spinal column with a forward concavity is known as lordosis. It occurs normally in the lower back region and is usually slightly more pronounced in females than in males. Slight lordosis is also present in the cervical area.

Curvature of the spinal column showing a backward convexity is called kyphosis and is normally present in the dorsal or upper back area.

Slight variations in the degrees of lordosis and kyphosis can and do occur quite normally but if these curvatures become exaggerated (or even at times reversed) then such a faulty posture will immediately cause strain and lead to further abnormalities if it is not corrected.

1. THE CERVICAL AREA

Throughout our whole life, practically all our everyday activities involve forward flexion of the head. The head and neck are bent forwards in eating, writing, reading and even resting on the pillow in bed. Very rarely do we look upwards and extend the head and neck backwards. Thus all our life the muscles at the posterior aspect of the neck are always being stretched. As we get older this leads to a weakness in this group of muscles. In chronic cases the patient can no longer pull his head backwards. Also in later life arthritic changes develop in the facet joints of the cervical vertebrae and osteophytic outgrowths develop in the opposing aspects of the vertebral bodies resulting in a lack of mobility in the cervical area.

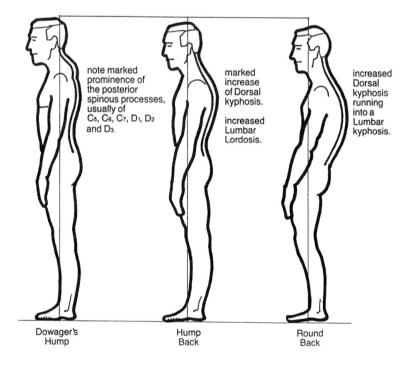

note marked prominence of the posterior spinous processes, usually of C_5, C_6, C_7, D_1, D_2 and D_3.

marked increase of Dorsal kyphosis.

increased Lumbar Lordosis.

increased Dorsal kyphosis running into a Lumbar kyphosis.

Dowager's Hump

Hump Back

Round Back

Thus with the onset of old age the head is commonly held forwards and its weight gradually flattens the normal cervical lordosis. In some cases this curve may even be completely reversed giving rise to cervical kyphosis. The flattening of the normal lordosis may extend as far as the upper Dorsal vertebrae and involve D.2 and D.3. It leads to the prominence of the posterior spinous processes, usually of C.5, C.6, C.7, D.1. and D.2. This condition is known as **'Dowager's Hump'** and usually, particularly in females, a pad of fat is superimposed over these processes.

Usually associated with this condition a rounding of the shoulders occurs, due to lack of tone in the posterior muscles of the shoulder joints.

2. **THE DORSAL AREA**

The constant pull forward of the neck upsets the normal alignment of the spinal column leading to a varying increase of dorsal kyphosis and if this becomes gross we refer to it as 'Dorsal Round Back', or 'Hump Back'.

3. **THE LUMBAR AREA**

If the muscle wasting process continues into the lumbar region, the normal lumbar lordosis decreases, giving rise to a marked reduction of the hollow in the lower back. In many cases, there is a complete reversal of the lumbar lordosis, producing a lumbar kyphosis. This deformity will join up with the dorsal kyphosis in the condition known as complete 'Round Back'.

4. **LOWER LIMBS**

At this stage the physical weight of the forward flexing of the head and upper dorsal regions puts a great strain on the weight-bearing joints of the lower limbs. In the complete 'round back' state the individual is now no longer able to regain the erect posture. As he is constantly fixed in forward flexion he may often fall forwards if his balance is seriously impaired. He will thus unconsciously seek to restore his balance by a slight forward flexion of the knee joints. In this condition great stress is exerted on these joints and this often leads to forward flexion of the lower end of the femur on the upper end of the tibia. With the onset of arthritis the ligaments may become overstretched, resulting in instability in the knee joints with the possibility of displaced cartilage. Fluid may collect around the joint and a good deal of pain will be present.

Walking with the back rounded and the knees bent forwards puts a tremendous strain on the hip joints. The weight of the trunk bearing down on these joints often causes the head of both the femur and that of the acetabulum to flatten and even, at times, the neck of the femur to bend downwards. This may cause an alteration in the angle of the joint articulation. This, in turn, causes the hip joints to splay outwards, resulting in an almost ape-like gait. Contraction of the surrounding ligaments and joint capsules is usually present in this condition.

The forward flexion of the knee joints not only disrupts the gait of the elderly person but increases the weakness of the lower limbs. Extra stress is exerted on the ankle joints. They become affected by the forward movement of the malleoli of the tibia and fibula on to the astragalus or talus leading to pain and swelling in the joints.

The whole weight of the trunk is now transferred to the feet. This leads to the condition of flat foot (Pes Planus) and results in added instability and diminished walking ability. In its simple form the two arches (the transverse or anterior arch extending under the metatarsal joints of the foot and the longitudinal arch extending from these joints to the os calcis of the heel) become flattened. The muscles, ligaments and tendons of the sole of the foot are stretched and the keystone of the arch of the foot (or astragalus) drops. Thus the 'spring' of the foot is lost and the patient adopts a marked shuffling gait.

These deformities obviously vary from individual to individual and are usually slower to develop in the healthy ageing person. They are nevertheless accepted by almost everyone as part of the normal process of growing old. I believe that such deformities can be prevented by a twice daily routine of the exercises described and illustrated in Part I. The specific training programmes I prescribe, are devised to prevent and/or correct the exaggerated forward flexion of the cervical (neck), dorsal (chest) and/or lumbar (lower back) regions of the spinal column. All these exercises act specifically on all muscles in the posterior aspect of the whole spinal column which may have lost their tone and power. Thus they tone in turn, all the muscles of the posterior cervical area, the posterior supra-scapular muscles, the posterior muscles of the shoulder girdle, all the muscles of the posterior dorsal area and finally all the muscles of the posterior or lumbar region. I have devised further exercises to tone up the muscles and joints of the lower limbs.

If a deformity has already begun to develop, **'surgical'**
manipulation may well be required to correct the abnormalities.
'Surgical' manipulation is a branch of surgery which has been
undeservedly neglected. It is so-called when practised by a fully
qualified medical person, but of course, involves no surgery in the
widely accepted sense of an operation. Partly, because of its neglect
by the medical profession, it has largely fallen into the hands of
unqualified practitioners. This is an unhappy situation — a real
misfortune — as 'surgical' manipulation, properly carried out on
suitable cases can be a most valuable therapeutic agent. 'Manipulative
surgery' aims at restoring normal movement which is commonly
absent in a stiff joint. A certain degree of **careful** force is always
necessary to correct joint alignment. Too much pressure or too
frequent treatments may result in reactionary painful swelling and
retard recovery. Usually 'surgical' manipulation is carried out twice
per week and the deformity corrected by the end of four weeks.
Thereafter, the patient must exercise rigorously and with perseverance
to tone up the muscles, that, most probably have begun to atrophy
from disuse, in order to gain full mobility of all the joints concerned.

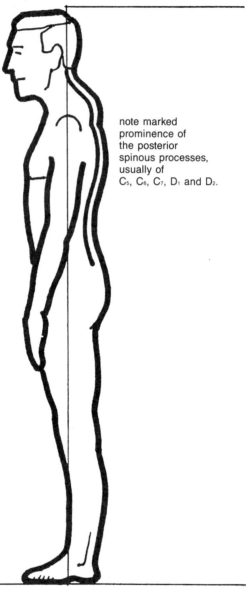

note marked
prominence of
the posterior
spinous processes,
usually of
C_5, C_6, C_7, D_1 and D_2.

Dowager's
Hump

88

CHAPTER THREE

Methods of Correcting the Deformities of the Spinal Column in the Aged

A. THE TREATMENT OF DEFORMITIES IN THE CERVICAL AREA

THE 'DOWAGER'S HUMP'

IN MOST cases, this condition starts to develop over the age of 40 and has been explained (see page 83) the cause of it usually, apart from trauma, or injury, is postural, for most every day actions, even sleeping, involve forward flexion of the head. The patient's occupation, if it involves bending the head forwards for long periods (for e.g. writers, surgeons etc.), may increase the tendency for this condition. Interestingly, it often has quite a distinct family background. It is fairly common for the patient to inform me that her mother, grandmother or an older sister has a similar deformity. I have examined older members of the family and some did have the deformity but in many cases, had no symptoms. It was quite interesting to note that the family in question appeared to have adopted the same postural habit.

Normally, in the lower cervical spinal area there is a slight to moderate forward angulation (cervical lordosis) at C.5/6/7/D.1, and the weight of the head is constantly bearing down on this angulation. As a result the posterior neck muscles at this level are liable to become overstretched and it is exactly at this level that the cervical or 'Dowager's Hump' develops. The facet joints may be pulled apart, with the overstretching of their intrinsic ligaments and muscles and as the condition progresses (especially in females) a layer of fat is often superimposed over these processes. Attacks of spondylitis and/or the onset of osteoarthritis may also cause changes in the surfaces of the joints and reduce mobility in this area. The normal lordosis of the cervical area becomes flattened and may even be reversed to show a cervical kyphosis.

Some patients, however, also show neurological symptoms, for example brachial neuritis or post occipital neuritis with headaches, which, at times have a migraine-like syndrome. In these cases a disc lesion is usually present. The precise diagnosis and treatment of such a lesion at any level in the cervical region is given in my recently published book.*

A lateral X-ray, if considered necessary, will usually show slight to moderage kyphosis, early spondylosis and early slight to moderate osteoarthritis. After the disc has been treated by my method of non-surgical detachment as described in my book,* 'surgical' manipulation is usually given to stretch the affected intrinsic muscles and ligaments. A training programme of exercises is prescribed. Such treatment also corrects the effects of early arthritis by rubbing one surface of the joint against the other until the surfaces become smooth and polished (eburnated) and thus move more easily and painlessly.

Where there is no disc lesion, and the condition is gross, 'surgical' manipulation may still be necessary. Thereafter, and in cases where the condition is still slight, I recommend the training programme as follows.

* 'The Slipped Disc and the Aching Back of Man'
by A. Walker-Naddell, published 1986 by J. R. Reid, Blantyre.

THE WALKER-NADDELL TRAINING PROGRAMME FOR CERVICAL AREA

Exercise I

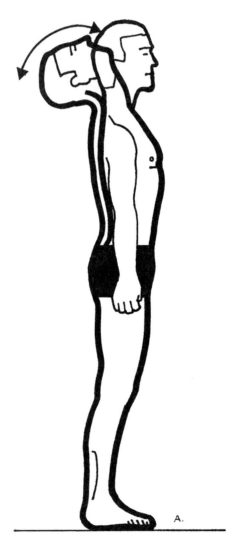

A.

THE WALKER-NADDELL TRAINING PROGRAMME
FOR THE CERVICAL AREA

Exercise I

1. Stand erect with feet slightly apart. Older patients may prefer to sit when doing Exercises I and II.

2. Jerk the head backwards, and then forwards but only as far as the erect posture, (never bending the neck forwards).

3. Repeat 10 times.

Exercise II

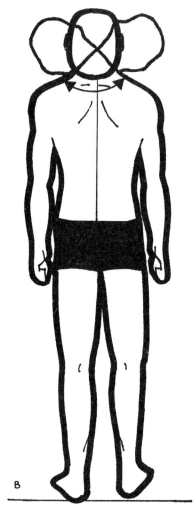

CERVICAL AREA

Exercise II

1. Stand erect with feet slightly apart.

2. Hold the head backwards.

3. Rotate the head in this axis, ear to shoulder, 10 times to one side and 10 times to the other side. Avoid bringing the head forwards beyond the shoulder point.

4. The rotation should follow the course of the round part of a capital 'D'. The head should never be rotated round and round as this will cause dizziness.

THE WALKER-NADDELL TRAINING PROGRAMME FOR CERVICAL AREA

Exercise III

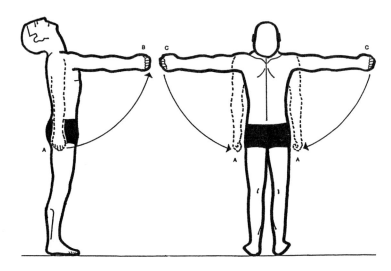

CERVICAL AREA

Exercise III

1. Stand erect with feet slightly apart.

2. Hold the head back, looking up to the ceiling.

3. Stretch the arms out straight in front and parallel to the floor.

4. With the elbow joints fixed and fists clenched rotate the stiff arms quickly backwards as if swimming breast stroke, with the shoulder blades coming together when the arms are right back.

5. Swing the stiff arms down past the body and repeat 20 times, four times a day. Take a deep breath when the arms are being raised to the horizontal plane, and exhale as the shoulder blades are brought together.

Exercise III, as well as getting the muscles of the neck in good tone, also exercises the supra-scapular, medial scapular and the arm muscles. If there is a degree of cervical spondylosis present, exercises II and III will tone up the affected muscles and ligaments and a full range of movement will be obtained.

THE WALKER-NADDELL TRAINING PROGRAMME FOR CERVICAL AREA

Exercise IV

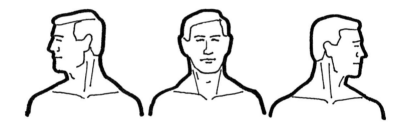

CERVICAL AREA

Exercise IV

1. The patient may sit or stand for this exercise.

2. With the head erect and looking forward, turn the neck slowly but firmly sideways, until the chin is in line with the top of the shoulder. Then pause for a count of five.

3. Perform the exercise five times in each direction, three or four times a day.

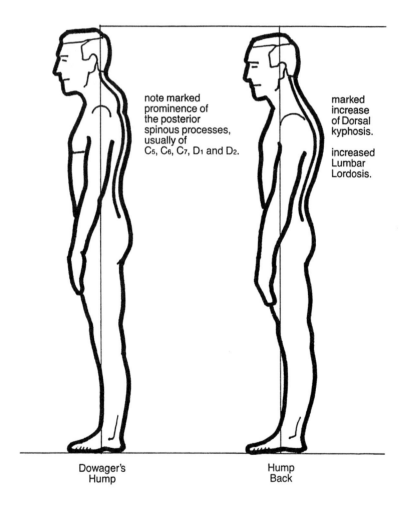

note marked
prominence of
the posterior
spinous processes,
usually of
C_5, C_6, C_7, D_1 and D_2.

marked
increase
of Dorsal
kyphosis.

increased
Lumbar
Lordosis.

Dowager's
Hump

Hump
Back

B. THE TREATMENT OF DEFORMITY IN THE DORSAL AREA — THE 'DORSAL ROUND BACK'

The 'Dorsal Round Back' develops as a progression of the condition of the 'Dowager's Hump'. The abnormal forward flexion of the neck gradually causes an increase in the normal dorsal kyphosis and when this becomes excessive it is called the 'Dorsal Round Back' or 'Hump Back'. As the condition progresses and the chest becomes flattened, it becomes increasingly difficult for the patient to take deep breaths. These are essential for the wellbeing of an active patient and a good supply of oxygen is necessary for muscle building. Diminished lung and chest movements leave the lungs susceptible to infection, thus varying degrees of bronchitis and even pneumonia may occur.

Patients may also show neurological symptoms and if this is the case a disc lesion in the dorsal area may be present. The diagnosis and treatment of a disc lesion at each level in this area is described in detail in my book* and usually surgical manipulation is also necessary.

When the condition is gross, even with no neurological symptoms, 'surgical' manipulation may often be required. It is also described in detail in my book.* Thereafter, and, also if the condition is not severe, I advise the patient to carry out the training programme I describe below. It is **vital** in this condition that the patient take deep breaths throughout the exercises, which should be done twice daily.

* 'The Slipped Disc and the Aching Back of Man'
by A. Walker-Naddell, published 1986 by J. R. Reid, Blantyre.

THE WALKER-NADDELL TRAINING PROGRAMME FOR DORSAL AREA

Exercise I

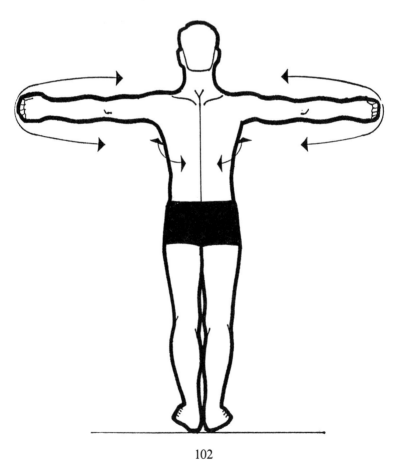

DORSAL AREA

Exercise I

1. Stand in the erect posture, with feet together, or slightly apart for extra stability.

2. With stiff elbow and wrist joints and clenched fists stretch the arms out sideways at shoulder level, parallel to the floor.

3. Holding this posture, whip the arms first one way and then the other, rotating the chest as far as it will go, from side to side. This, in turn, rotates the dorsal or thoracic vertebrae.

4. Repeat 20 times in each direction, four times a day.

5. Breathe in and out with each movement.

THE WALKER-NADDELL TRAINING PROGRAMME FOR DORSAL AREA

Excercise II

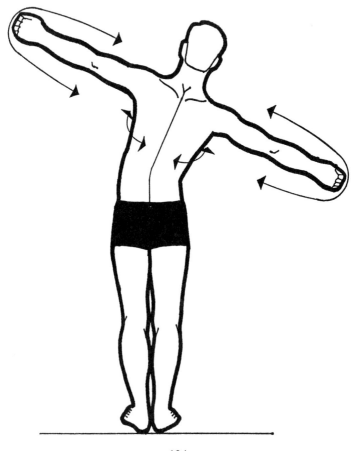

DORSAL AREA

Exercise II

1. Stand in the erect posture with feet together, or slightly apart for extra stability.

2. With stiff elbows and wrist joints and clenched fists stretch the arms out sideways at shoulder level, parallel to the floor.

3. Lower one arm, bending at the waist with the other pointing upwards, still with the arm straight and in line with the tip of the shoulders.

4. Holding this posture, whip the arms first one way and then the other.

5. Repeat 10 times in each direction.

6. Repeat 10 further times with the chest flexed at the waist in the opposite direction.

7. Inhale and exhale regularly to prevent overtiring of the muscles.

THE WALKER-NADDELL TRAINING PROGRAMME FOR DORSAL AREA

Exercise III

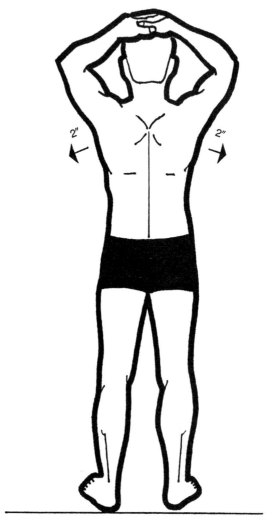

DORSAL AREA

Exercise III

1. The patient may either sit or stand.

2. Clasp hands on the top of the head, with elbows raised as high as possible.

3. Swing the chest from side to side for about 2″, extending upwards with every movement.

4. Repeat 20 times in each direction.

THE WALKER-NADDELL TRAINING PROGRAMME FOR DORSAL AREA

Exercise IV

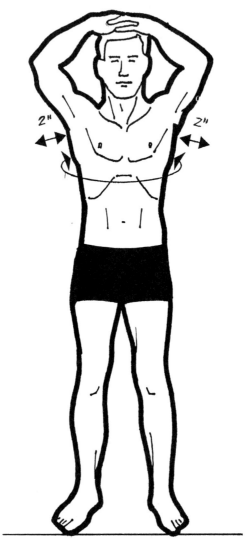

DORSAL AREA

Exercise IV

1. Adopt the same posture as for Exercise III.
2. Rotate the chest, bending 2″ in all directions.
3. Repeat 20 times one way and 20 times the other.

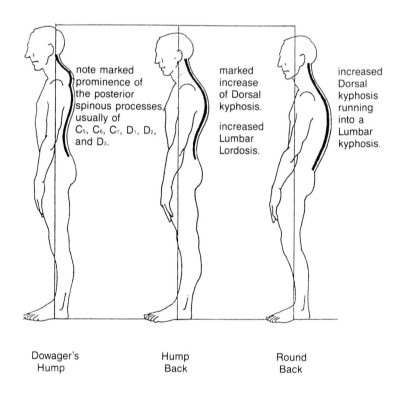

note marked prominence of the posterior spinous processes, usually of C_5, C_6, C_7, D_1, D_2, and D_3.

marked increase of Dorsal kyphosis.

increased Lumbar Lordosis.

increased Dorsal kyphosis running into a Lumbar kyphosis.

Dowager's Hump

Hump Back

Round Back

C. **THE TREATMENT OF DEFORMITY IN THE LUMBAR AREA — THE COMPLETE ROUND BACK**

The increased dorsal lordosis present in the condition of the 'Dorsal Round Back' or 'Hump Back' may extend into the lumbar area. The normal Lumbar lordosis becomes increased, producing the 'Complete Round Back'.

Patients suffering from neurological symptoms should be referred for possible diagnosis and treatment of a disc lesion in the lumbar area. My book*, describes in detail the treatment of all cases, including sciatica and lumbago.

'Surgical' manipulation is usually necessary in these cases and may also be required if the condition is gross though showing no neurological symptoms. During this course of treatment, and afterwards, the patient should perform the set of exercises described below, twice daily.

* 'The Slipped Disc and the Aching Back of Man'
by A. Walker-Naddell, published 1986 by J. R. Reid, Blantyre.

THE WALKER-NADDELL TRAINING PROGRAMME FOR THE LUMBAR AREA

Exercise I

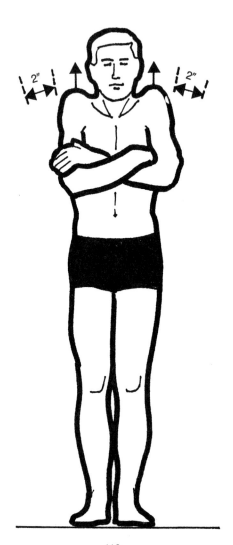

LUMBAR AREA

Exercise I

MUSCLE TONING TRACTION

1. Stand erect with feet together, or slightly apart for extra stability.

2. Expand chest, this increases lumbar curve.

3. Fold arms across chest.

4. Raise points of shoulders to ears.

5. In this posture move the chest for 2″ from side to side 25 times each way, bending through waist.

6. Take a deep breath with each movement. The shoulders should remain fixed in this position. It is the chest which moves from side to side and at the same time it is being pulled upwards all the time.

THE WALKER-NADDELL TRAINING PROGRAMME FOR LUMBAR AREA

Exercise II

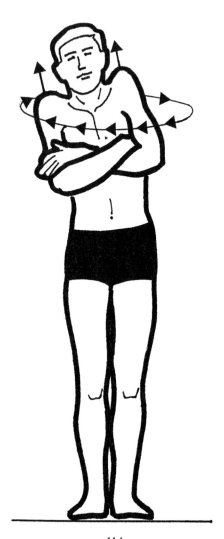

LUMBAR

Exercise II

MUSCLE TONING TRACTION WITH SPINAL ROTATION

1. Adopt the same posture as in Exercise I.

2. Rotate the chest through the waistline round and round for no more than 2″ from the vertical — first 20 times in one direction and then 20 times in the other direction.

THE WALKER-NADDELL TRAINING PROGRAMME FOR LUMBAR AREA

Exercise III

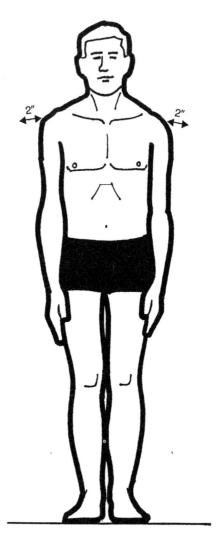

LUMBAR AREA

Exercise III

PENDULUM MOVEMENT OF THE TRUNK

1. Stand in the erect posture with the arms kept at the side of the body.

2. Keep the chest expanded, which increases the lumbar lordosis.

3. Flex the chest laterally 25 times from side to side, 2″ in either direction at speed. Bend at waist only. Do not move legs. The shoulders are held fixed and only move with the chest.

THE WALKER-NADDELL TRAINING PROGRAMME FOR LUMBAR AREA

Exercise IV

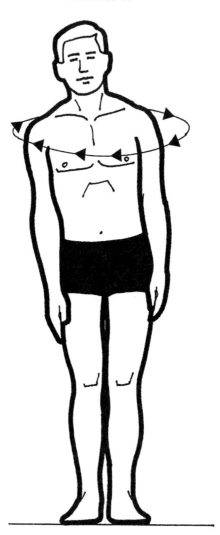

LUMBAR AREA

Exercise IV

ROTATION OF THE TRUNK THROUGH THE WAIST LINE

1. Stand in the erect posture as in Exercise III.

2. Rotate the chest, bending at waist line only, not more than 2″, 25 times in one direction and 25 times in the other.

3. Arms kept close to body.

4. Shoulders are not raised, but move with the chest.

THE WALKER-NADDELL TRAINING PROGRAMME FOR LUMBAR AREA

Exercise V

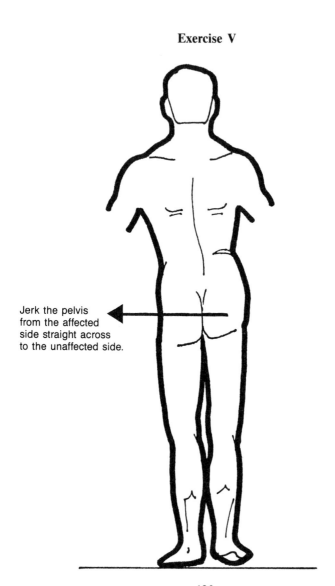

Jerk the pelvis from the affected side straight across to the unaffected side.

LUMBAR AREA

Exercise V

PELVIC JERK

Jerk the pelvis from the affected side straight across to the unaffected side, i.e. from right to left (for a right sided scoliosis), 20 jerks four times per day.

SHOULDER JOINT

Frontal Section through the Right Shoulder Joint.

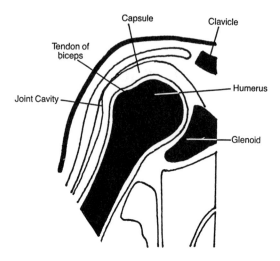

Capsule
Clavicle
Tendon of biceps
Humerus
Joint Cavity
Glenoid

Vertical sections through the shoulder joint, the arm being vertical (above)
and (below) with the arm parallel to the ground.

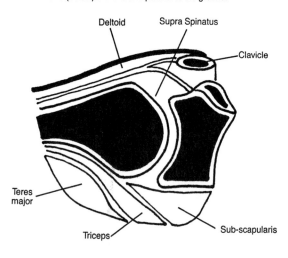

Deltoid
Supra Spinatus
Clavicle
Teres major
Triceps
Sub-scapularis

CHAPTER FOUR

The Treatment of the Deformities of Specific Joints in the Aged

THE natural slowing down process of old age, together with possible osteoarthritis, not only affects the spinal column, producing the distinctive posture associated with the elderly and the problems that arise from these postural deformities, but it also often causes deformities in specific joints. In the dorsal area, the shoulder joint is often affected and, in the lumbar area, the hip and knee joints are particularly vulnerable.

A. THE SHOULDER JOINT

The shoulder joint is a ball and socket joint formed by the large globular head of the humerus articulating with the much smaller, shallow articular surface of the glenoid fossa of the scapula. It appears to be a poorly designed joint, permitting very considerable movement. To avoid displacement it relies on all the tendons and muscles of the shoulder girdle that surround it, to a much lesser degree on the capsule that surrounds the joint and to the shoulder joint ligaments. The capsule is relatively loose to provide for the unusual freedom of movement normally present in this joint.

As one gets older, there is usually a slowing down process. The physical movement of the muscles diminishes and may lead to disuse atrophy of certain or all of the muscles. The shoulder joints tend to fall forward as the muscles in the dorsal area lose tone, causing a drooping and rounding of the shoulders. Varying degrees of loss of movement occur in one or both shoulder joints and give rise, in more severe cases, to the condition known as **FROZEN SHOULDER or CUFF SYNDROME.**

This condition may also occur as a result of injury, such as a fall on the shoulder or a stretch pull of the joint. Thus, in these cases, it can occur in much younger patients but, regardless of age or cause,

SHOULDER JOINT

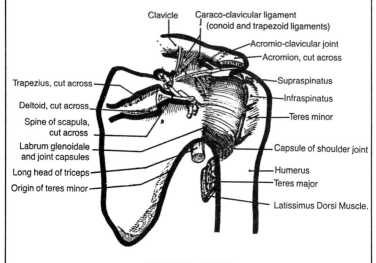

Clavicle

Caraco-clavicular ligament
(conoid and trapezoid ligaments)

Acromio-clavicular joint

Acromion, cut across

Trapezius, cut across

Supraspinatus

Infraspinatus

Deltoid, cut across

Teres minor

Spine of scapula,
cut across

Labrum glenoidale
and joint capsules

Capsule of shoulder joint

Long head of triceps

Humerus

Origin of teres minor

Teres major

Latissimus Dorsi Muscle.

POSTERIOR ASPECT
(DEEPER DISSECTION)

the treatment of frozen shoulder is carried out in exactly the same manner. In cases due to trauma, the capsule of the joint is stretched and as most of the muscles of the shoulder pass through the capsule they too become affected.

In all cases it is of the utmost importance once a firm diagnosis has been reached that treatment is undertaken immediately to prevent a chronic state of affairs setting in. When this happens, the damaged capsule contracts, thus restricting the muscle movement which passes through it. Adhesions form between the muscle and the capsule and may lead to a disuse atrophy of the affected muscle.

The severity of the condition will vary from individual to individual depending on the duration of the complaint and the initial cause. In all cases a varying degree of loss of movement is present in one or both joints and any attempt at further movement is always accompanied by acute pain. The patient will have difficulty in raising his arm on the affected side: even in bringing his hand to his mouth when eating and excessive movement when dressing may also cause acute pain. Such everyday activities may be associated with both pain and frustration.

TREATMENT

The condition is treated by instructing the patient to carry out a specific routine programme of exercises. These involve a variety of shoulder movements which basically are designed to regain tone in the muscle groups and, at the same time, gradually to stretch the capsule of the shoulder joint.

In cases of frozen shoulder I avoid manipulation whether by local anaesthetic or by using a general. Whereas it would be relatively simple to stretch the joint by manipulation, such treatment may result in the tearing of the contracted capsule and possible tearing or overtearing of the affected muscle groups. It must also be noted that the muscles are not in tone and until they are they have not got the power to move or control the shoulder joint after manipulation. Thus the important factor is gently to exercise the muscles in order to tone and strengthen them.

THE WALKER-NADDELL TRAINING PROGRAMME FOR FROZEN SHOULDER OR CUFF SYNDROME

Patients are warned that during this training programme they must never go through the point of pain. This would possibly damage tissue and retard their progress. They should do the exercises regularly and systematically but always stop before the point of pain. Gradually, but surely, the extent of movement will increase. Whereas possibly at the first consultation, the patient may not be able to raise his arms up to shoulder level, at the second or third visit he may raise his arms as far as his mouth and at the fourth up to his eyes. Finally full movement of the arms up to the head will be achieved.

Patients are also asked to carry out the programme using both arms. In past experience I noted that invariably a patient who had recovered from one frozen shoulder returned later with the condition affecting the opposite shoulder. I can give no anatomical reason for this. However, I have discovered that if the patient trains both shoulders the condition does not develop in the unaffected joint.

THE WALKER-NADDELL TRAINING PROGRAMME FOR THE SHOULDER JOINT

Exercise I

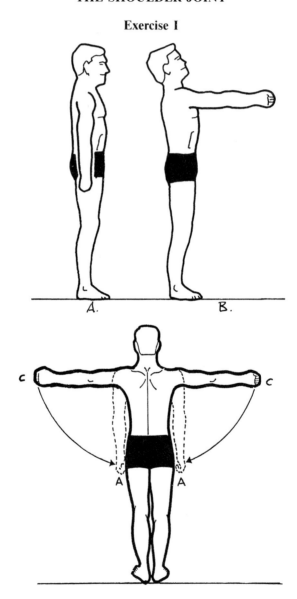

THE SHOULDER JOINT

Exercise I

1. Stand erect, with feet slightly apart.

2. With clenched fists and stretched taut arms raise the arms from the side of the body forwards and upwards, just short of the point of pain.

3. From this position (and it may not even be at shoulder level) move the arms round in a breast stroke movement, round and back to the sides of the body.

4. This should be done 20 times.

THE WALKER-NADDELL TRAINING PROGRAMME FOR THE SHOULDER JOINT

Exercise II

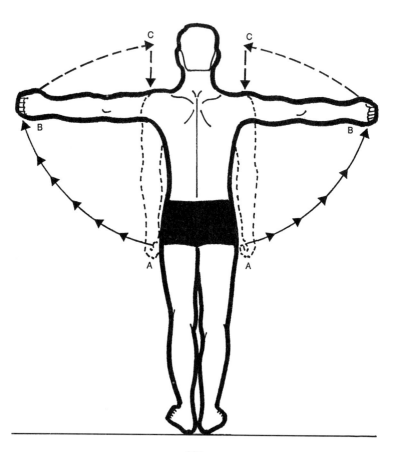

THE SHOULDER JOINT

Exercise II

Reverse the rotation of Exercise I, holding the same position, and moving the arms backwards at the level without pain and rotating forwards until the hands are to the side of the body again. This should be done 20 times.

Day by day and very gradually the patient will notice that the level, to which he can lift his arms without pain to begin the exercise, will be raised.

THE WALKER-NADDELL TRAINING PROGRAMME FOR THE SHOULDER JOINT

Exercise III

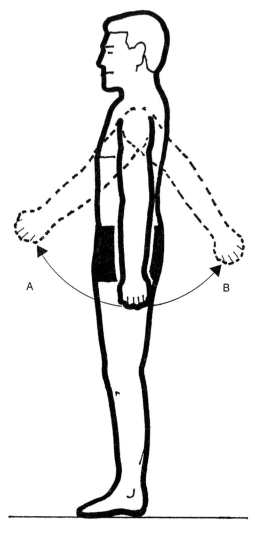

THE SHOULDER JOINT

Exercise III

1. Adopt the same position as in I and II with clenched fists and arms like rods.

2. Swing the arms parallel to the sides of the body forwards and backwards, as far as possible **without** pain.

3. This should be done 20 times.

THE WALKER-NADDELL TRAINING PROGRAMME FOR THE SHOULDER JOINT

Exercise IV

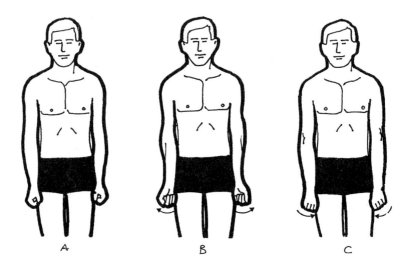

A   B   C

THE SHOULDER JOINT

Exercise IV

1. Adopt the same position as in I, II and III with the fists clenched and the arms taut.

2. Hold the arms close to the sides of the body and rotate the upper arms, one way and then the other, using a screwdriver type of action, as if 'driving' the screw into the ground.

3. This should be done 20 times.

This training programme is demonstrated to the patient at the first consultation. I ask him to return about four days later to make quite sure that the routine is being carried out properly. Invariably, I find that the patient has been over zealous in one movement or another and, despite my instructions, has attempted to go through the point of pain and has thus retarded the recovery process.

I usually see the patient four times over a period of one month and at each consultation I assess the degree of mobility of the joint. During the examination I support the affected arm with one hand under the elbow joint of the extended arm and, with the other hand resting on the superior aspect of the shoulder joint, I raise the whole arm upwards until I reach the point of pain. I can easily assess the increase of mobility in the joint by assessing the extent of the angle of the arm to the body. I lower the arm still supporting it at the elbow joint as soon as the point of pain has been reached.

In my experience all traces of a frozen shoulder which I have treated as described are usually completely cleared up at the end of one month, provided that the patient conscientiously carries out the training programme, and once the condition has cleared away, it never returns.

THE ELBOW JOINT

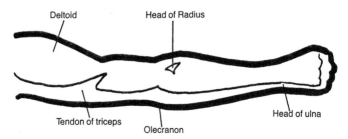

Surface Landmarks on the Back of Upper Limb.

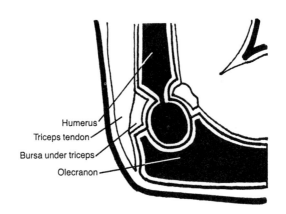

Vertical Section through the Elbow Joint.

B. THE ELBOW JOINT

The condition known as 'TENNIS ELBOW' commonly affects the elderly though this condition, as its name suggests, can affect all age groups. The treatment is the same for young and old and has proved very satisfactory in all cases though, as is usual, the earlier the diagnosis, the more quickly the condition will clear up.

The elbow joint is a hinge-joint and formed by the articulation of the humerus with the greater sigmoid cavity of the ulna and the lesser or radial head of the humerus with the cup-shaped depression on the head of the radius. The rotation movement at the elbow is obtained by the articulation of the circumference of the head of the radius with the lesser sigmoid cavity of the ulna i.e. the radio-ulnar articulation that allows movement of rotation of the radius on the ulna. The articular surfaces are covered by a thin layer of cartilage and connected together by a capsular ligament that varies in thickness. The thickened portions are usually described as four distinct ligaments: the anterior, the posterior, the internal lateral and the external lateral.

The condition of tennis elbow is caused by uric acid crystals forming between the radius and the lower end of the humerus. I believe that trauma may also be responsible for the onset of this condition. Injury may cause the jarring of one bony surface against the other and this may lead to damage of the surfaces and the flaking of the hyaline joint surfaces. The patient will suffer acute pain with any joint movement and be very susceptible to any external contact with or pressure on the joint.

THE ELBOW JOINT

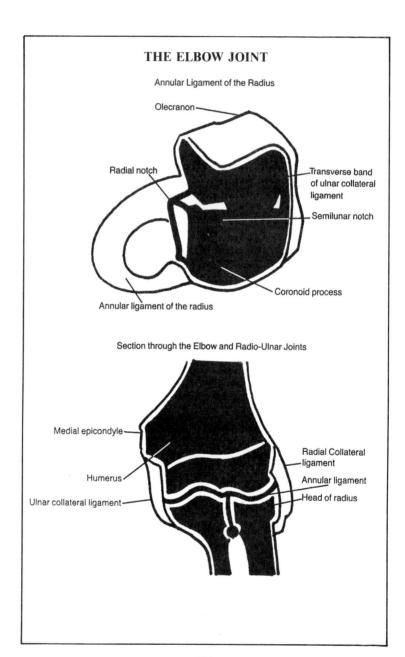

Annular Ligament of the Radius

Olecranon

Radial notch

Transverse band
of ulnar collateral
ligament

Semilunar notch

Coronoid process

Annular ligament of the radius

Section through the Elbow and Radio-Ulnar Joints

Medial epicondyle

Radial Collateral
ligament

Annular ligament

Humerus

Head of radius

Ulnar collateral ligament

THE TREATMENT OF TENNIS ELBOW

After diagnosis I usually manipulate the elbow at the first consultation. I inject a small quantity of local anaesthetic into the capsule of the joint at the affected side. After a few minutes I compress firmly at the joint articulation to expel any uric acid crystals which may be formed in the joint capsule.

Then I demonstrate the exercise that I instruct the patient to carry out as often as possible during the day.

THE WALKER-NADDELL TRAINING PROGRAMME FOR TENNIS ELBOW

Exercise

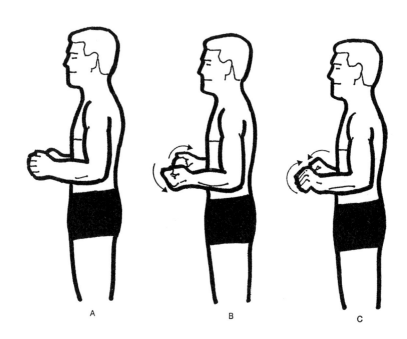

A   B   C

TENNIS ELBOW

Exercise

1. The patient may sit or stand but the latter is perhaps preferable.

2. The arms should be bent at the elbows to form a right angle.

3. The fists should be clenched at all times and the wrists kept straight with the forearm.

4. Holding the upper arms firmly in to the side of the body the forearms should be rotated through the elbow joints slowly and firmly, first one way and then the other 20 times.

THE WRIST JOINT

Vertical section through the articulations at the wrist, showing the five synovial membranes.

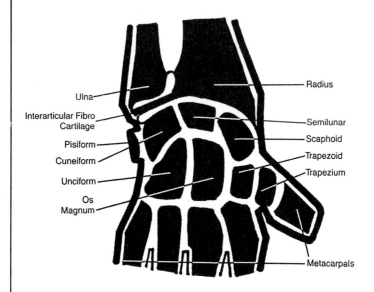

Ulna

Interarticular Fibro Cartilage

Pisiform

Cuneiform

Unciform

Os Magnum

Radius

Semilunar

Scaphoid

Trapezoid

Trapezium

Metacarpals

C. **THE WRIST JOINT AND THE FINGER JOINTS**

The wrist joint is formed by the lower end of the radius articulating with the carpal bones, or more precisely, the scaphoid, the semi-lunar and cuneiform bones. Between the lower articulating end of the radius and these carpal bones lies the interarticular fibro-cartilage. The remaining five carpal bones take no part in the formation of the wrist joint. All the bony surfaces of the articulation are covered with cartilage and are connected together by a capsule.

In old age the commonest injury to the wrist joint is fracture through the thinning waist of the scaphoid bone. This thinning is caused by the presence of slight osteoporosis that often affects the elderly (see Appendix). Arthritis in the wrist joint also occurs in the elderly, preventing mobility of the joint. At times, a gross lack of rotation and loss of dorsi and palmar flexion (up and down movement) is experienced on account of the pain involved.

TREATMENT

The fracture of a scaphoid in an elderly person is best treated by putting a light crepe bandage around the wrist as this permits some degree of movement. If plaster of paris is used to immobilise the joint a gross disuse atrophy normally ensues and recovery from this state of affairs rarely occurs.

I recommend that the training exercises set out below be carried out with the bandage still in place to keep the joint gently mobile and prevent atrophy of surrounding muscles.

Patients who are suffering from arthritis of the wrist joint(s) are asked to follow the same training programme.

THE WALKER-NADDELL TRAINING PROGRAMME FOR THE WRIST JOINT

Exercise I

Rotation

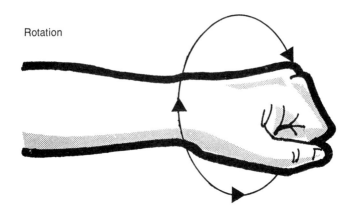

Rotation in reverse

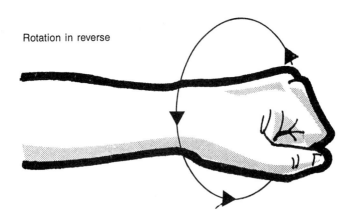

THE WRIST JOINT

Exercise I

1. The exercise may be done sitting or standing.

2. Bend the arm at the elbow and keep the arm taut. Hold the arm into the side of the body.

3. Rotate the hand through the wrist joint, five times in one direction and five times in the opposite direction.

4. This exercise should be carried out at least four times a day.

THE WALKER-NADDELL TRAINING PROGRAMME FOR THE WRIST JOINT

Exercise II

Dorsi Flexion.

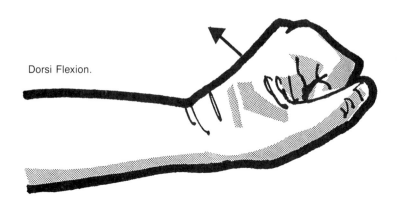

Palmar Flexion.

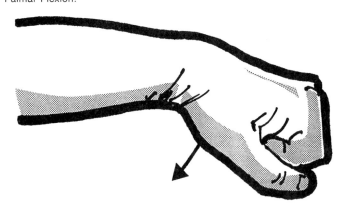

THE WRIST JOINT

Exercise II

1. Adopt the same position as for Exercise I.
2. Bend the hand up and down from the wrist with fist clenched — 10 movements in all, five up and five down.

FINGER JOINTS

Stiffening of the finger joints is very common in the elderly and thus dexterity may be grossly impeded. To prevent this, older people should exercise the fingers in the following way.

Exercise I

Flex the fingers up and down in sequence, as if playing the scales on a piano.

Exercise II

Stretch the hand in order to separate the fingers as far as possible and hold the hand in this position for a minute, or say, for a count of 20.

THE HIP JOINT

Oblique Section through Right Hip Joint.

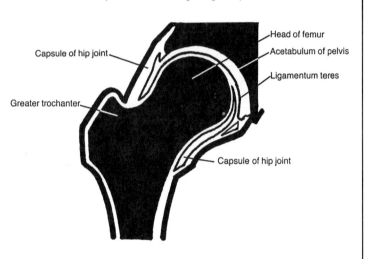

Capsule of hip joint

Greater trochanter

Head of femur

Acetabulum of pelvis

Ligamentum teres

Capsule of hip joint

Left hip joint laid open.

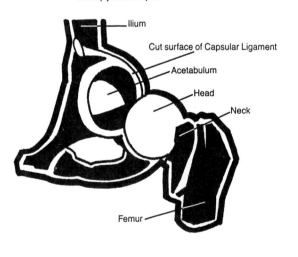

Ilium

Cut surface of Capsular Ligament

Acetabulum

Head

Neck

Femur

Methods to Prevent and Correct Deformity of the Lower Limbs

D. THE HIP JOINT

THE hip joint is a 'Ball and Socket' joint, in which the head of the femur normally fits snugly into the acetabulum, which is part of the pelvis. This joint is as notable for its strength as the shoulder joint is for its weakness. It has a much smaller range of movements and activity than the shoulder joint and dislocation of the joint is extremely rare. The action of gravity holds the bones together and surrounding the joint are powerful ligaments and very strong masses of muscles.

The frequent lack of mobility in the elderly often causes the muscles to become weak with overstretching of the ligaments around the joint, and gradually the space between the head of the femur and the acetabulum to become narrowed. This narrowing results in flattening, both of the femoral head and also that of the acetabulum. To prevent subluxation of the hip joint in these conditions, the rim of the acetabulum often becomes thickened.

The hip joint is the largest of the weight-bearing joints of the lower limbs. The weight of the trunk bearing down on the joint also contributes to the flattening of the head of the femur and of the acetabulum. This pressure may also cause the neck of the femur to be bent downwards, giving rise to coxa vara. The varying degrees of flattening of the femoral head commonly causes the capsule of the hip joint to contract and possibly some alteration of the angle of the neck of the femur occurs. This may lead to a varying degree of limp with loss of the joint movement, associated with pain. This process can also result in a reduction of the patient's height of up to 1½″. The alteration of the angle of articulation of the joint also causes the head and the neck of the femur to splay outwards and the patient often adopts a waddling or ape-like gait.

Varying degrees of arthritic change often takes place in the hip joints in the elderly, resulting in a degree of crepitus (creaking) in the affected joints. Mobility can be grossly affected, depending whether one or both joints are affected. The change caused by this arthritis is due in many cases to the laying down of uric acid crystals on the opposing joint surfaces, though injury is certainly a predisposing factor for the onset of this condition.

Pain and a limp are two of the commonest symptoms in arthritis of the hip joint condition. The pain and limp are due to a roughening of the surfaces of the two segments of the ball and socket joint, causing one surface, as it were, to spike into the other. The important factor of the treatment of arthritis of the hip joint is to eradicate the cause of the patient's symptoms by giving the patient a specific training programme. The use of these exercises causes one rough surface of the joint to run against the other and the uric acid crystals in the joint to be broken off and ultimately absorbed. This treatment can be compared with the rubbing of two pieces of sandpaper, one against the other. If this is done constantly the 'spikes' on the sandpaper will wear off and the surfaces become smooth. Similarly in the joint, the opposing surfaces will become polished or eburnated and mobility in the joint will be regained.

It is vitally important for the surgeon to keep in mind that the earlier he attacks this problem the more quickly the patient will become mobile; the disease will be arrested and there will be no further deterioration of the bone surfaces. Thus replacement joints in hip surgery would no longer be necessary in the majority of cases.

Decalcification, associated with osteoporosis often occurs in the joint and is treated by a course of calcium with vitamin D, together with the use of a training programme, as described earlier and in the Appendix.

ASSESSMENT AND TREATMENT OF HIP JOINT DEFORMITY

Before commencing treatment and setting out a training programme for the patient I always assess the degree of restriction of movement in the affected joint. I ask the patient to sit in an upright chair in the surgery with his sacrum well back against the back of the chair. I raise in turn each knee joint towards the patient's chest and can assess the degree of joint movement present in either or both hip joints. If there is no abnormality in the joint the thigh will almost press against the anterior chest wall. This provides the yardstick to gauge any restriction of joint movement.

Then the patient is asked to lie on his back on the orthopaedic couch, with his legs bent at the knee joints. The legs are bent upwards towards the anterior chest wall. Again if the hip joints are normal (or if one is normal) the knee or knees can be easily pressed against the chest wall. If this is not possible one can easily assess the degree of arthritis present in that joint. Audible creaking will also be present in the affected joint. While the patient is still lying on his back, I ask him to bend his legs at the knee joints and pull them up until the thighs are at approximately right angles to the trunk and the soles of the feet flat on the couch. Then the knees are pulled apart to assess the amount of mobility present. In an affected joint the movement will be restricted and painful, but very slowly and gently I pull the limb outwards a little further in order to stretch the contracted joint capsule. With the patient still in this position I hold the knee joint and rotate the hip joint in both directions, stopping just short of the point of pain. This not only stretches the posterior aspect of the joint capsule but it also rubs one rough surface of the joint against the other, thereby smoothing the joint movement.

At this stage I ask the patient to move over to the edge of the couch until he lines up the middle of his sacrum with that edge. I push the knee down towards the floor. This hyperextends the hip joint. If there is full movement in the joint there will be no restriction or pain but if abnormality is present the capsule will be stretched, producing pain.

X-rays are now taken to ascertain the degree of deformity that has occurred in the structure of the bones of the joint.

Then I explain in detail the exercises of a Training Programme that I advise my patients to carry out regularly and with enthusiasm, for by doing so they will speed up their own recovery. The exercises in most cases simulate the gentle manipulation I have given at the time of assessment, and will give at all subsequent consultations. If the Training Programme is carried out faithfully, restriction of joint movement will diminish and full movement will eventually be achieved without any further pain.

THE WALKER-NADDELL TRAINING PROGRAMME FOR THE HIP JOINTS

Exercise I

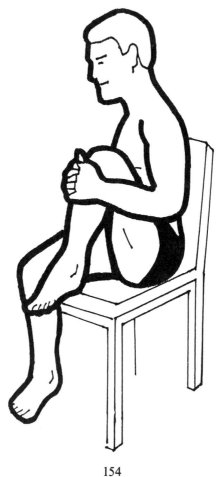

THE HIP JOINT

Exercise I

1. Sit well back in an upright chair. Clasp hands in front of the knee joints and pull the knee joints up. Press the knee joints as far as possible towards the chest and hold for a count of five. This will stretch the capsule of the hip joints.

THE WALKER-NADDELL TRAINING PROGRAMME FOR THE HIP JOINTS

Exercise II

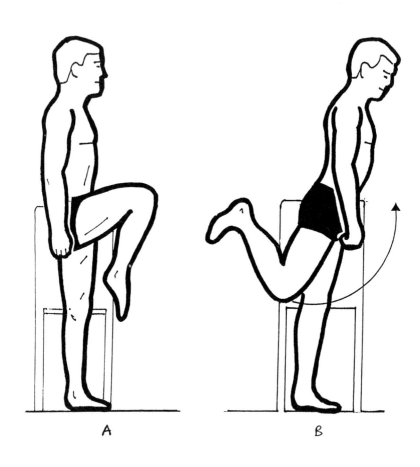

A   B

THE HIP JOINT

Exercise II

1. Stand at the side of a strong chair holding the back of it with one hand. Bend the opposite leg at the knee joint so that the lower leg is at right angles to the thigh.

2. Swing the leg backwards and forwards, ensuring the leg is still bent. This should be done 20 times with each leg.

THE WALKER-NADDELL TRAINING PROGRAMME FOR THE HIP JOINTS

Exercise III

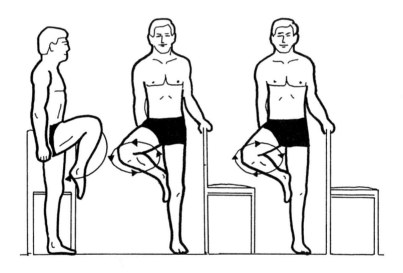

THE HIP JOINT

EXERCISE III

1. Adopt the same position as in Exercise II with the leg still bent at right angles.
2. Rotate the leg from the hip joint, 20 times one way and then 20 times the other, exercising each leg in turn.

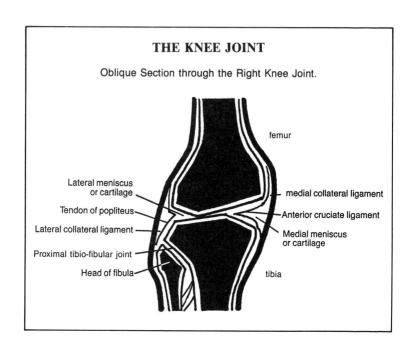

THE KNEE JOINT

Oblique Section through the Right Knee Joint.

femur

Lateral meniscus or cartilage

Tendon of popliteus

Lateral collateral ligament

Proximal tibio-fibular joint

Head of fibula

medial collateral ligament

Anterior cruciate ligament

Medial meniscus or cartilage

tibia

160

E. THE KNEE JOINT

The knee is primarily a hinge joint, though slight rotary movement is also present. It is formed by the articulation of the lower end of the femur with the upper end of the tibia, with the medial and lateral cartilages intervening.

It should always be borne in mind that the knee joint has no muscles of its own. It relies on the muscles of the anterior part of the thigh: i.e. the quadriceps group and the tibialus articus below the knee. If these muscles, particularly the quadriceps lose their tone the knee joint becomes vulnerable and easily injured. The ligaments of the joint are the two cruciates and the medial and lateral collateral ligaments. The commonest injury to the knee joint is the overstretching of the ligaments, in particular the medial collateral ligament, and this gives rise to an unstable knee joint. A sudden twist of the knee joint laterally, say from walking or running over rough ground, could cause a fall and overstretching of the medial collateral ligament. Because this ligament has the medial cartilage attached to it, this sudden lateral twist could easily tear the outer rim of this cartilage, giving rise to a condition commonly called a 'Bucket-handled tear' of the medial cartilage or meniscus. It produces marked swelling of the joint, the fluid of which is, at times, haemorrhagic. Footballers and rugby players are prone to this type of injury. Fortunately the lateral collateral ligament is not attached to the cartilage, so a 'bucket-handled tear' never occurs if injury is experienced there.

In the ageing process the forward flexion of the head and the rounding of the back in a forward direction (see Diagram on page 76) puts a tremendous strain on the knee joints which are bent forward by the patient in order to retain the erect posture. This results in an often gross defective walking movement. As a result of this and the possible onset of arthritis the movement of the lower limbs becomes slow and possibly painful. Muscle wasting will set in and often the arches of the feet will flatten and toe deformities develop.

The bending forward of the knee joints frequently adopted by the elderly to regain their balance and prevent themselves falling forward often causes the lower end of the femur to slide forward on the upper end of the tibia and results in varying degrees of stretching of the patellar ligament. This produces an unstable joint and to prevent subluxation of the joint, thickening occurs in the bone ends which form the joint i.e. the lower end of the femur and the upper end of the tibia.

THE KNEE JOINT

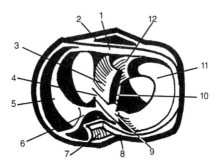

The Menisci and their Attachments

1. Transverse ligament.
2. Anterior cornu of medial meniscus.
3. Anterior cruciate ligament.
4. Medial tubercle of intercondyloid eminence of tibia.
5. Medial meniscus.
6. Posterior cornu of medial meniscus.
7. Posterior cruciate ligament.

8. Fasciculus from lateral meniscus to posterior cruciate ligament.
9. Posterior cornu of lateral meniscus.
10. Lateral tubercle of intercondyloid eminence of tibia.
11. Lateral meniscus.
12. Anterior cornu of lateral meniscus.

Stretching of all the ligaments of the knee joints commonly occurs as a result of an awkward gait and once again this causes the joint to become unstable. In these conditions any slight twist, particularly laterally, may lead to a 'bucket-handled' tear of the medial cartilage or meniscus. Thus the cartilage problem may affect the elderly almost as commonly as the sportsman.

Onset of arthritis in the knee joint commonly occurs as one gets older and creaking (or crepitus) is evident during movement of the joint.

ASSESSMENT AND TREATMENT OF ARTHRITIS OF THE KNEE JOINT

If the knee joint appears to be grossly arthritic i.e. badly swollen and giving a good deal of pain, I arrange X-rays to be taken of both joints to assess the extent of the condition. Because the patient is suffering a great deal of pain, I read these plates immediately so that treatment may begin at that consultation. In order to reduce the swelling commonly present in the joint I aspirate the fluid from it. This is done under local anaesthesia. A few drops of local anaesthetic are injected under the skin at the affected site and the fluid is drawn off using either a trochar and cannula or even a simple wide-bored needle. This treatment may have to be repeated once or twice more.

As the knee is a weight-bearing joint I always advise my patients to rest as much as possible, cutting down walking to an absolute minimum.

Once the fluid has been completely and finally removed, examination usually reveals that the capsule of the knee joint, particularly at its posterior aspect has contracted.

163

THE WALKER-NADDELL TRAINING PROGRAMME FOR THE KNEE JOINTS

Exercise I

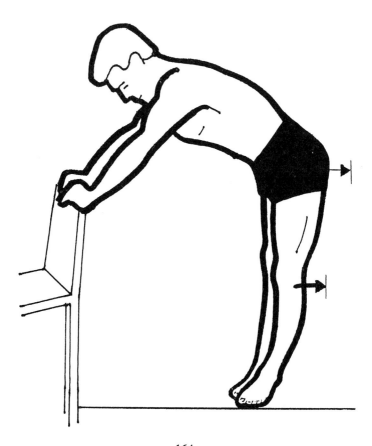

THE WALKER-NADDELL TRAINING PROGRAMME
TO CORRECT DEFORMITY IN THE KNEE JOINTS

At this stage I prescribe a training programme for the patient to carry out. If he adheres to it faithfully he will help himself to make a speedy recovery. The programme aims to correct the forward bending of the knee joint and at the same time to tone up the quadriceps and tibialus groups of muscles. It is designed to make the three corrections in one specific group of exercises.

THE KNEE JOINTS

Exercise I

1. Stand behind a strong high-backed chair about a foot away from it.

2. Rest the hands on the back of the chair.

3. Rise up on the toes and pull the knee joints backwards as far as possible.

4. Bend the trunk towards the top of the chair, without touching it, still ensuring the knee joints are pulled backwards. Hold in this position initially for a count of 10 and later for 20.

THE WALKER-NADDELL TRAINING PROGRAMME FOR THE KNEE JOINTS

Exercise II

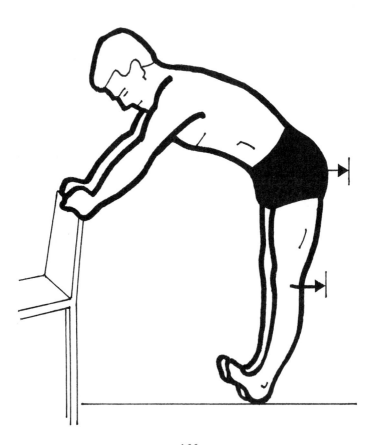

THE KNEE JOINTS

Exercise II

1. Adopt the same attitude as for Exercise I, again resting the hands on the back of the chair and standing about a foot behind it.

2. Rise up on the heels, with toes pointing towards the chin.

3. Pull the knee joints backwards as far as possible despite the pain involved.

4. Bend the chest towards the top of the chair without touching it, still pulling the knee joints backwards, regardless of pain and hold for a count of 10 initially, and later for 20.

I assess the progress the patient has made with the Training Programme and if I feel that further treatment is required I then manipulate.

The Manipulation

The patient is asked to lie on his back on the orthopaedic couch. I inject two or three drops of local anaesthesia into the capsule of the joint on both sides of the patella. After about five minutes I place one hand just above the knee joint and the other just under the calf, pushing the femur down with one hand and pulling the tibia up with the other. One commonly hears audible clicks as the adhesions that have formed are broken down.

I carry out this manoeuvre each time I see the patient and usually after about four treatments the knee joint is quite straight.

TREATMENT OF DISPLACED CARTILAGE

In cases with displaced cartilage I assess firstly whether excess fluid is present within the joint. If it is, then I aspirate immediately to reduce the swelling. While the local anaesthetic is still effective, the patient is asked to lie on his back on the couch. If say, the medial cartilage has been displaced, I put one thumb on the cartilage. I place the other hand on the patient's ankle and bend the leg laterally. At the same time as I push the cartilage in I jerk the leg laterally and upwards towards myself.

I then recommend patients to follow the Training Programme described above. The elderly must follow this programme with perseverance to tone up the muscles that are often either lacking in tone or atrophied.

This complaint is a common one amongst **footballers** and they usually sustain a 'bucket-handled' tear of the cartilage. As described above I aspirate immediately if the joint is swollen under local anaesthetic and replace the cartilage by manipulation under the same local anaesthesia. Though the footballer is asked to adopt the same Training Programme as the elderly it must be remembered that footballers are athletes with muscles in perfect tone and thus they will not need to follow the programme for very long before the condition has settled down. Usually they can play football again within two weeks.

However, in young or old, it is important to realise that cartilage tears will heal and it is beneficial for all to keep the muscles above and below the knee joint in such good tone that the joint will not be unstable and thus easily prone to injury.

THE ANKLE JOINT

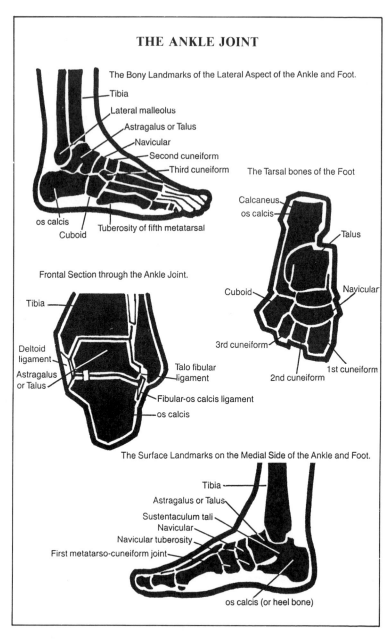

The Bony Landmarks of the Lateral Aspect of the Ankle and Foot.

Tibia

Lateral malleolus

Astragalus or Talus

Navicular

Second cuneiform

Third cuneiform

The Tarsal bones of the Foot

os calcis

Cuboid

Tuberosity of fifth metatarsal

Calcaneus
os calcis

Talus

Cuboid

Navicular

3rd cuneiform

2nd cuneiform

1st cuneiform

Frontal Section through the Ankle Joint.

Tibia

Deltoid ligament

Astragalus or Talus

Talo fibular ligament

Fibular-os calcis ligament

os calcis

The Surface Landmarks on the Medial Side of the Ankle and Foot.

Tibia

Astragalus or Talus

Sustentaculum tali

Navicular

Navicular tuberosity

First metatarso-cuneiform joint

os calcis (or heel bone)

F. THE ANKLE JOINT

The ankle joint is a hinge joint. It is formed by the lower extremity of the tibia and its malleolus and the external malleolus of the fibula which articulate with the upper convex surface of the astragalus or talus and its two lateral facets. The astragalus occupies the middle and upper part of the tarsus, supporting the tibia above and resting upon the os calcis or heel bone, that lies below it. The bony surfaces are covered with cartilage and connected together by a capsule, which in places forms thickened bands constituting four ligaments: the anterior, the posterior, the deltoid or internal lateral and the external lateral.

The two malleoli serve as important guides in the region of the ankle joint. The lateral malleolus which is the distal end of the fibula is the larger of the two and its tip is a ¼" below the level of the medial malleolus, and ¾" behind it. The medial malleolus is itself the distal end of the tibia. Sited between these bone ends is the astragalus (or talus) bone, thus forming the ankle joint. This bone is significant, for it forms the keystone of the longitudinal arch of the foot and bears to a considerable degree the weight of the whole body in the erect position. The tibio-fibular mortice is shaped to fit the upper articular surface of the talus or astragalus which is broader in front than behind.

In old age when flat foot often develops (see next section) this keystone or astragalus (or talus) is compressed downwards, forwards and medially and the interval between it and the tuberosity of the os calcis (heel bone) is enlarged. In time this leads to a distinct prominence on the medial border of the foot, in front of the medial malleolus and causes overstretching of the soft tissues on the sole of the foot i.e. the plantar muscles, the ligaments and the joint capsules. This condition is known as static flat foot.

In further old age when the elderly tend to bend the knee joints forward to maintain the erect posture, greater strain is exerted on the ankle joints. In this posture the malleoli of the tibia and fibula, bearing the whole weight of the body, are pushed forwards. This in turn puts great backward pressure on the ankle joints, particularly pushing the talus and os calcis backwards which in turn pulls the whole foot backwards. This together with the onset of arthritis which causes some deformity in these joints, often results in a subluxation backwards of the ankle joint.

THE ANKLE JOINT

Tendon sheaths on front of ankle.

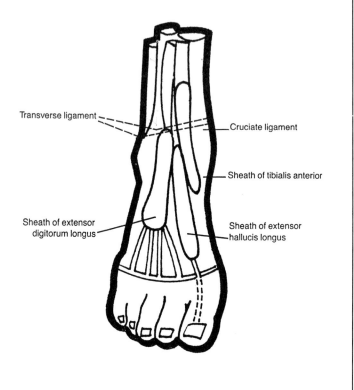

Transverse ligament

Cruciate ligament

Sheath of tibialis anterior

Sheath of extensor digitorum longus

Sheath of extensor hallucis longus

SYMPTOMS

1. Moderate to severe pain in the region of the ankle joint which is aggravated in the acute phase by movement.

2. Swelling below the malleoli of the ankle joint is commonly present with some swelling, as a rule, in the region of the astragalus (or talus) bone, just below the medial malleolus.

3. The astragalus bone, which is the keystone of the longitudinal arch of the foot, usually drops downwards and medially giving rise to a bony prominence just below and in front of the medial malleolus. The whole foot then becomes everted. This is a common feature in static 'flat foot'.

4. All associated ligaments become stretched, particularly the deltoid which runs from the medial malleolus to the astragalus and on to the os calcis.

TREATMENT

The ankle should be rested initially but the exercises described below should be performed, gently at first, even while resting in bed or sitting in a chair.

THE WALKER-NADDELL TRAINING PROGRAMME FOR THE ANKLE JOINT

Exercise I

Dorsi Flexion of the Ankle Joint.

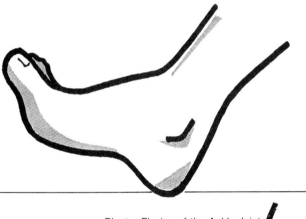

Plantar Flexion of the Ankle Joint.

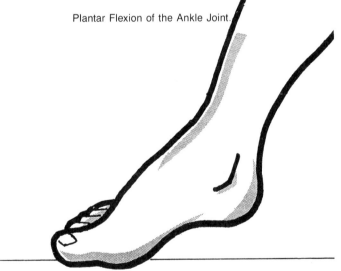

Extension and Flexion of the Ankle Joint.

THE WALKER-NADDELL TRAINING PROGRAMME FOR ANKLE DEFORMITY

Exercise I

The ankle joint should be flexed up and down 20 times exercising each foot in turn. Initially it should be carried out four times a day.

THE WALKER-NADDELL TRAINING PROGRAMME FOR THE ANKLE JOINT

Exercise II

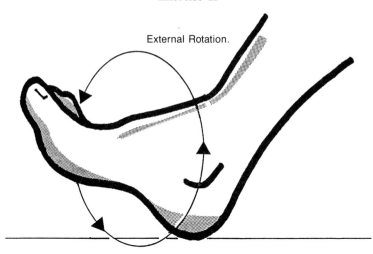

External Rotation.

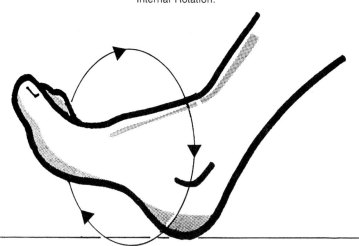

Internal Rotation.

Rotation of the Ankle Joint.

THE ANKLE JOINT

Exercise II

Rotate the ankle joint, first inwardly 20 times and then in the opposite direction 20 times, exercising each foot in turn.

These movements prevent the formation of bony adhesions, contraction of the ligaments and gradually they will tone up the muscles which control the ankle joint movements.

THE WALKER-NADDELL TRAINING PROGRAMME FOR THE ANKLE JOINT

Exercise III

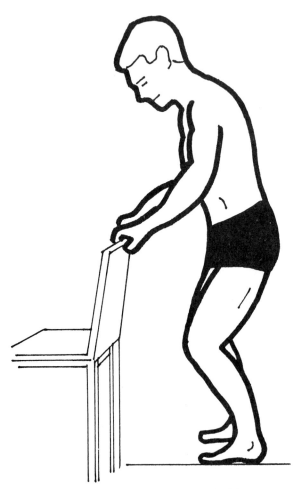

Exercise for Dorsi Flexion of the Ankle Joints.

THE ANKLE JOINT

Exercise III

1. Stand behind a strong dining chair and hold the back with both hands.
2. Feet should be about a foot behind the chair, flat on the ground.
3. Bend the knees forwards as far as possible with the feet still remaining flat on the floor.
4. Hold in this position for a count of 10 later 20.

TREATMENT BY SURGICAL MANIPULATION

The above movements of these exercises are carried out by the surgeon increasing the range with each effort. In most cases the astragalus or talus bone has dislocated downwards and medially. This must be reset into its correct position by everting the forefoot with one hand and firmly pressing the astragalus or talus bone laterally and upwards into its correct position. This deformity takes time to clear up. With treatment once a week it may take as long as six months. If one attempts to treat these cases too frequently, there is every likelihood of reactionary swelling and pain occurring in the region of the ankle and this would, of course, retard recovery. Full recovery can be achieved with patience and perseverance.

THE FEET

The normal plantar print of the sole of the feet.

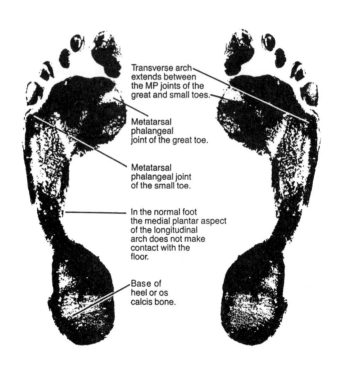

Transverse arch extends between the MP joints of the great and small toes.

Metatarsal phalangeal joint of the great toe.

Metatarsal phalangeal joint of the small toe.

In the normal foot the medial plantar aspect of the longitudinal arch does not make contact with the floor.

Base of heel or os calcis bone.

G. ASSESSMENT AND TREATMENT OF THE DEFORMITIES OF THE FEET

The entire body weight is supported by the foot. In bearing heavy weights or jumping from a height the extra strain is taken by the foot. The human foot has become highly specialised to support the weight of the body under the changing conditions imposed upon it by various human activities. In its static or passive function it supports the body weight of a person when standing, with stability over lengthy periods. When a person is walking or even more so when running, in addition to providing at each step a stable base for the temporary support of the body weight, it must at the same time be sufficiently pliable and resilient to provide a spring or lever by which the body can be propelled forwards. This function is often lost in old age with the flattening of the foot arches and deformities arising in the tarsal and metatarsal bones. The 'spring' of the step is lost and the elderly adopt a shuffling gait.

To fulfil the requirements made of the foot a kind of elastic structure has developed made up of a great number of little bones held together by ligaments, tendons and muscles. These form the transverse and longitudinal arches.

Two powerful tendons act as most important 'slings' for the support of the longitudinal arch; they are the tendons of the peroneus longus and tibialis posterior.

THE LONGITUDINAL ARCH

This extends from the base or plantar surface of the os calcis forwards to the metatarso-phalangeal joints of the forefoot. It consists of inner and outer portions, resting on a common pillar posteriorly — the tuberosity of the os calcis or calcaneus. The inner part of the longitudinal arch is formed by the astragalus or talus, the navicular, the three cuneiform bones, and the inner three metatarsals and corresponding phalanges. The outer part of this longitudinal arch is formed by the os calcis or calcaneus, the cuboid, the outer two metatarsals and their corresponding phalanges.

THE FEET

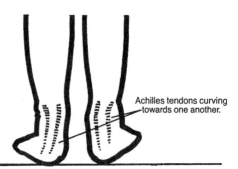

Achilles tendons curving towards one another.

Flat Foot Deformity of the Feet as seen from behind.

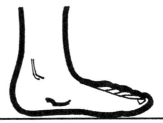

Flat Foot with dropped Longitudinal Arch and Prominence of the Navicular. The rigid type.

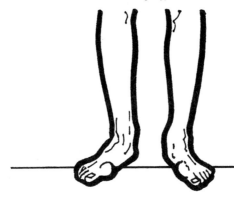

Flat Feet with Bunions.

The astragalus or talus is the KEYSTONE of the arch. It receives the body weight and transmits it to the arches below. Pressure is exerted on three points: the base of the os calcis at the heel forms one and the other two are at the base i.e. the plantar aspects of the first and fifth metatarso-phalangeal joints of the great and small toe respectively. These three points form an important tripod maintaining balance. This can be disturbed when the head of the first metatarsal is removed in the bunion operation.

When standing erect the inner border of the foot is straight or concave. When the arch collapses as in flat foot, this concavity becomes a convexity because the head of the talus projects down into it.

TRANSVERSE OR ANTERIOR ARCH

This extends from the base or plantar aspect of the small toe across to the base or plantar aspect of the great toe.

The metatarsal and tarsal bones are arranged in a convex curve on the dorsum and a concave arch on the plantar aspect of the foot.

FLAT FOOT OR PES PLANUS

The condition of 'Flat Foot' may arise under many circumstances but they have one effect in common — they create a disproportion between the load on the arch of the foot and the structures supporting it. Flat foot may be caused by an abnormal distribution of the body weight on the arch when, for example, the foot has assumed an everted posture. Long periods of standing or fatigue may result in loss of tone in the leg muscles and may further result in flattening of the arches of the feet. A rapid increase in body weight and a return to activity after a long illness are two other causes of flat foot.

Flat foot is also a very common condition in the elderly. During the ageing process there is often a tendency to bend the head forward with a rounding of the shoulders. This forward flexion may continue until the whole trunk is bent forwards. In order to prevent the person falling forwards and to try and maintain an erect posture, the knee joints are bent forwards. Walking with forward flexion of the knee joints puts a great strain on these joints, with overstretching of the ligaments and in many cases, displacement of the cartilage. Great strain is exerted in the ankle joints which, in turn, distorts the tarsal joints. Various deformities of the feet result — in particular the flattening of the arch of the feet.

THE FOOT

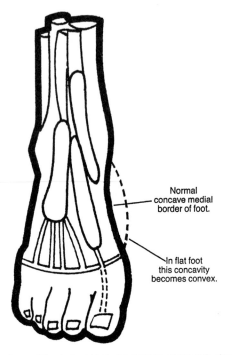

Normal concave medial border of foot.

In flat foot this concavity becomes convex.

In flat foot the talus bone of the foot, which is the keystone of the arch, drops downwards and medially. Thus the concavity of the forefoot becomes convex, with flattening of the long arch of the foot.

SYMPTOMS

In the flat foot (or pes planus) the two arches of the foot, the longitudinal and the transverse, are lost and the plantar aspect of the foot is flat. During the flattening process the ligaments, tendons and muscles supporting the arch become stretched and inefficient and the astragalus is no longer supported and drops. The astragalus bone, rather like the keystone of a bridge, is the 'keystone' of the longitudinal arch. When the astragalus drops, it forces its way between the internal malleolus and the tubercle of the scaphoid. It may actually touch the ground. The result of this condition is that the forefoot is deflected laterally. Eversion of both the sole of the foot and the mid-tarsal joint occurs and the inner margin of the sole of the foot becomes depressed and the outer margin raised. The original concavity of the inner foot becomes decidedly convex in the flat foot condition.

Eventually in neglected cases, i.e. when the spinal or joint deformities are not corrected, the bones of the foot may become distorted by osteophytic outgrowths and the astragalus or keystone of the arch may be ankylosed. Thus the 'spring' of the arch is completely lost.

TREATMENT

When I examine the feet of the patient it is not difficult to recognise the flattening of the foot arches and thus the condition of the flat foot. It is important to assess the degree of flattening in the arch by specific tests.

To check the state of the **longitudinal arch** I ask the patient to stand behind a high-backed chair. I then ask him to rise up on his toes and still in this position to separate the heels, keeping the great toes together, and to lean towards the chair. Not only does this allow the consultant to assess the ability to raise the longitudinal arch but this test also forms a basis for treatment. The patient is asked to do this every hour and remain in this position for a count of up to 20.

To check the state of the **anterior arch,** I ask the patient to stand on a piece of paper covered with chalk. If the anterior arch is normal then only the metatarso-phalangeal (MP) joints of the great and small toes will touch the paper. If, however, the arch is flat all the MP joints of the three remaining joints will also be flat on the paper. The degree of flattening can be easily assessed by this simple method.

185

Initially, correction of the flattening of the anterior arch is carried out by manipulation. The forefoot is held firmly with one hand and each MP joint, in turn, is held between the thumb and forefinger of the other hand and gently flexed downwards i.e. plantar-side. Audible clicks will be heard. These are due to the breaking down of adhesions as these joints, as a rule, have become arthritic.

The patient is asked to do this similarly at home i.e. plantar flexion of all the toes, one at a time, counting up to five with each toe. Regular use of this training exercise will regain the transverse arch of the foot, although it may take months depending on the age of the patient, the severity of the condition and the degree of deformity.

I also advise them to do the following exercises to restore the longitudinal arch in particular.

THE WALKER-NADDELL TRAINING PROGRAMME FOR THE ARCHES OF THE FEET

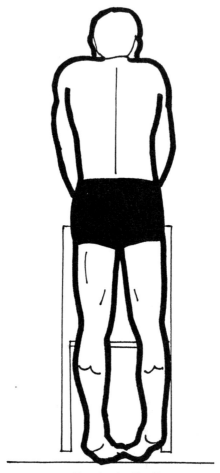

Exercise for Flat Feet.

ANTERIOR ARCH

The exercises for the ankle joint will also tone the muscles of this arch if the toes are curled downwards.

LONGITUDINAL ARCH

Exercise I

1. Stand behind a high backed chair, about a foot behind it and hold the back of the chair with both hands.

2. Rise onto toes as high as possible, with feet together.

3. In this position separate both heels as far as possible, keeping great toes together.

4. Hold this position for a count of 20.

BUNION DEFORMITY OF THE FOOT (Hallux Valgus)

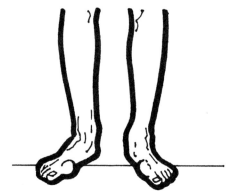

Flat Feet with Bunions.

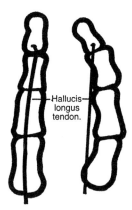

Hallucis longus tendon.

Diagram of the 1st metatarsal joint of the great toe, showing on the right, bunion deformity.

DISABILITIES WHICH ENSUE AS THE RESULT OF THE FLAT FOOT CONDITION

When the arches of the foot are lost the conditions listed below often follow or are associated with flat foot. This is an excellent illustration of how alteration of the anatomical angles of the foot may produce a whole chain of deformities. These are:

1. Hallux Valgus

2. Hammer Toe

3. Hallux Rigidus

4. Hallux Flexus

1. **HALLUX VALGUS** (Bunion)

The great toe should point straight forward in line with the long axis of the first metatarsal bone. When the arches of the foot are lost, the forefoot i.e. the tarsal bones may be displaced and the great toe may be bent laterally. As the angle of the great toe, articulating with the metatarsus has become distorted the small muscles inserted into the base are now acting at a mechanical disadvantage, and they pull the great toe further laterally. The line of pull of the long extensor tendon, (hallucis longus), instead of being along the line of the first metatarsal and the big toe, now acts along a line external to that and still further increases the deformity. A bunion commonly forms over the medial aspect of the metatarso-phalangeal joint which becomes swollen and extremely painful. The bursa at the MP joint becomes inflamed and the slightest pressure on the affected joint gives rise to such pain that it becomes difficult to put on a pair of shoes or even slippers. Thus mobility is greatly diminished and a marked disuse atrophy of the joint and muscles sets in.

Food and drink also play an important role in the formation and aggravation of the bunion condition. I recommend that patients avoid taking an excess of sugar and most alcoholic drinks, especially wine.

In flat foot the talus bone of the foot, which is the keystone of the arch, drops downwards and medially. Thus the concavity of the forefoot becomes convex, with flattening of the long arch of the foot. The normal alignment of the tendon of the great toe (hallucis longus) is displaced laterally, pulling the base of the first phalanx in which it is inserted also laterally. This, in turn, bends the great toe itself laterally, **thus increasing the bunion deformity.**

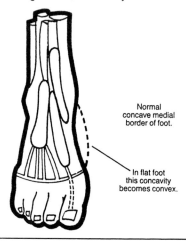

Normal
concave medial
border of foot.

In flat foot
this concavity
becomes convex.

TREATMENT

In acute cases the patient is advised to rest the foot as much as possible. Walking becomes almost impossible on account of the severe pain in the great toe and it would only aggravate the condition. In these cases I insert a toe separator in the form of a rubber splint between the great and second toes.

I ask the patient to keep the splint in position and move around normally for no more than two hours and then to remove it. The following day he should use it for a period of three hours and thereafter for a whole morning or afternoon. Once the condition has settled down the toe flex should be washed and kept safely away so that the same method of usage can be carried on in the event of a further attack. I always advise my patients to avoid using tight-footed stockings or socks or wearing pointed shoes as these only lead to a cramping or bunching of the toes laterally. If a patient is bunion-prone he or she, should always wear broad-fitting shoes — this is not always acceptable to ladies who often prefer to suffer a little discomfort for the sake of fashion! They should, however, limit the wearing of a stylish shoe to about three hours.

HAMMER TOE

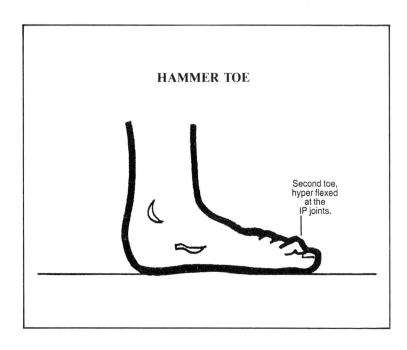

Second toe,
hyper flexed
at the
IP joints.

2. HAMMER TOE

The displacement of the great toe outwards in the condition of Hallux Valgus (Bunion) causes the other toes to become cramped for room in the shoe and as a result, one of the toes usually the second, is displaced forwards. It becomes acutely flexed at the first interphalangeal joint. The bones forming this joint thus form a prominence and constant chafing and pressure of a shoe on the joint often causes a corn to develop. The point of the last phalanx may press against the shoe sole and also result in a corn. The pressure of the shoe in these circumstances causes extreme pain and thus mobility is impaired.

TREATMENT

The hammer toe condition is corrected initially by manipulation. One hand holds the forefoot firmly whilst the other hand holds the affected toe with the thumb of that hand placed over the dorsal aspect of the MP joint which is affected and the forefinger placed underneath the joint. I then straighten the joint by firm flexion of my thumb towards my index finger under the toe.

I instruct the patient to carry out this training programme at home as many times a day as possible and to return for a final check-up at the end of one month.

3. HALLUX RIGIDUS

With the onset of arthritis that commonly affects the elderly, the metatarso-phalangeal joint of the great toe is often affected, resulting in pain and eventually a lack of movement in the joint. In chronic cases in which the arthritis of the MP joints is acute a moderate degree of arthrodesis sets in and the joint becomes rigid. In this condition the great toe is in a line with the first metatarsal. There is usually thickening of the metatarso-phalangeal of the great toe with pain in attempting flexion or extension of this joint. It is a common complaint in footballers and in people who wear shoes which although broad fitting are too short for the foot, thus the MP joint of the great toe is constantly being stubbed.

TREATMENT

An attempt to correct this condition is by gentle manipulation, which may be increased to two or three times a week if there is no immediate reaction. Plantar and dorsi flexion of the MP joint as described earlier for the correction of the anterior arch, is carried out gently. The patient is asked to do this exercise at home as often as is possible and to return to me in approximately one month.

In order to immobilise the joint and prevent excess strain on it during every day activities I recommend that a shoe maker inserts a small steel plate between the two flat layers of leather of the sole of the shoe, extending the whole length from the top of the toe to just beyond the whole length of the first metatarsal bone. This prevents plantar and dorsi flexion of the great toe.

4. HALLUX FLEXUS

Arthritis in the foot often causes the long extensor tendon, which is attached to the dorsal aspect of the first phalanx, to become overstretched and adhere to the arthritic joint. The plantar tendons remain unaffected and pull the great toe downwards, giving rise to the condition known as Hallux Flexus. In this condition the great toe cannot be extended but remains permanently flexed towards the sole of the foot.

TREATMENT

The correction of the Hallux Flexus is carried out initially by manipulation. As the great toe is literally hanging downwards, I place the thumb of one hand on the plantar aspect of the terminal phalanx and the index finger of the same hand on the dorsal aspect of the MP joint. I hold the forefoot firmly in the other hand and then push firmly upwards with my thumb in order to correct the deformity. Here again the patient is asked to carry out this treatment at home and hold the toe upwards and backwards for a count of 20 each time. This should be done three times a day. As arthritis is usually present in the MP joint audible clicks and crepitus will be noted. If the conditions fails to clear up by the end of one month, a special plantar splint is made for the patient. A metal plate is inserted into the sole of the shoe which keeps the great toe extended. In time the arthritic MP joint surfaces will adhere to one another and the patient will be left with a moderate degree of Hallux Rigidus.

A number of colleagues prefer to open up the MP joint and if the damaged tendon cannot be fixed to the phalanx, arthrodesis is carried out i.e. the surfaces of the MP joint are removed. This may shorten the toe and occasionally arthrodesis fails. In this case the patient may unfortunately be left with a flail joint.

OSTEOPOROSIS

Photograph of part of the spinal column showing marked decalcification and distortion of the bodies of the vertebrae in osteoporosis.

Vertebral
Bodies

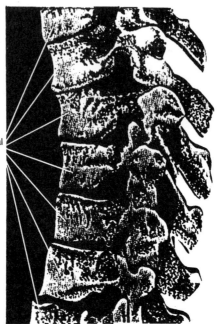

Osteoporosis

OSTEOPOROSIS is a chronic degenerative condition of the bone, which results in an abnormal porousness or rarefaction of bone causing enlargement of its canals or the formation of abnormal spaces.

The bones of the body form the main structures of the body and act as scaffolding for the attachment of the muscles that maintain the correct alignment of the skeletal system and permit locomotion. The skeletal system provides protection for the vital organs, such as the brain, heart, spinal cord etc. Most importantly, the bones of the body also act as a storage reservoir for various essential minerals, particularly calcium.

Bone formation is not static throughout all our lives. In youth it is required for growth when bones are lengthening and the young person is growing taller. It is important therefore to ensure that a diet containing an adequate amount of calcium be given during this growing phase. An insufficiency of calcium can produce a variety of bony deformities like rickets, knock-knees or bowing of the knees etc. Once the bones have reached adult proportions no further actual growth takes place but the make-up of the bone is constantly changing. Throughout life minerals in the bone tissue are being deposited by the osteoblasts and removed by the osteoclasts. In normal adults the amounts of bone formation and bone resorption are equal but in old age the bone formation often becomes less than bone resorption. The bone mass tends to decrease and the bones become osteoporotic.

OSTEOPOROSIS AND THE AGEING

It is now generally accepted that the ageing process is associated with bone loss and the onset of osteoporosis and the latter appears to affect more women than men. In a careful study of 500 cases suffering from osteoporosis my series revealed that 75% were females

OSTEOPOROSIS

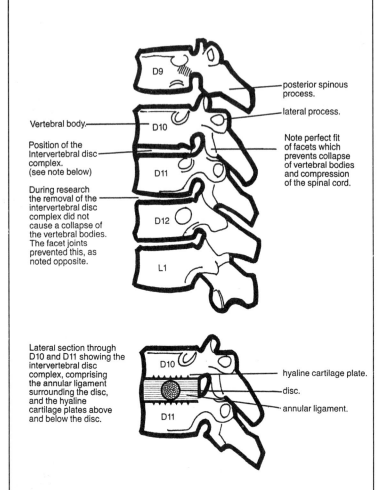

D9

posterior spinous process.

lateral process.

Vertebral body.

D10

Position of the Intervertebral disc complex. (see note below)

Note perfect fit of facets which prevents collapse of vertebral bodies and compression of the spinal cord.

D11

During research the removal of the intervertebral disc complex did not cause a collapse of the vertebral bodies. The facet joints prevented this, as noted opposite.

D12

L1

Lateral section through D10 and D11 showing the intervertebral disc complex, comprising the annular ligament surrounding the disc, and the hyaline cartilage plates above and below the disc.

D10

hyaline cartilage plate.

disc.

annular ligament.

D11

Schematic presentations showing articulation of the facet joints in a segment of the spinal column and the position of the intervertebral disc complex.

and only 25% males. From collected evidence there seems no doubt that the onset of the menopausal syndrome due to hormonal imbalance has a direct bearing on the onset of osteoporosis. This has been confirmed to some extent by the discovery that osteoporosis can affect some very young women athletes. The vigorous training that they undergo often results in menstrual cycle irregularities, or amenorrhoea. It suggests that the hormonal imbalance that gives rise to amenorrhoea is also responsible for the onset of osteoporosis. It seems obvious, therefore, that some hormonal therapy is called for, but to avoid the various possibly adverse side effects only a very small dose of oestrogen, administered weekly, should be given.

The word 'osteoporosis' simply means the development of a porous structure in bone. The remaining bones become thin and brittle and the slightest blow can lead to a fracture, or even several fractures, with gross deformity often resulting. The treatment of these cases is extremely difficult because there is often a failure of bony union. The patient may become bedridden and immobile with a marked ongoing gross disuse atrophy of muscles. Immobility in fact, plays an important role in the development of osteoporosis. This has now been convincingly demonstrated in bedrest and space flight simulations under research conditions.

Osteoporosis, however, in fact, attacks only a certain type of bone, and that is cancellous bone. Most of the bones in the human body are made up of compact bone, but cancellous bone is present in the vertebral bodies of the spinal column and small quantities are also present in other areas, such as the metacarpal bones of the hand and the tarsal bones of the feet. Osteoporosis is thus a fairly common back condition that particularly affects the older age groups, especially people over 60 years of age. Normally it rarely affects the younger age groups. It gives rise to back pain and usually a deformity at the affected site. The lumbar and dorsal regions of the spine are the areas most commonly involved but any part of the spinal column may become affected.

When osteoporosis develops in the spinal column it affects only that part of the vertebra that is medically known as the 'body' of the vertebra. This is composed of cancellous tissue, covered by a thin layer of compact bone as distinct from the other bony parts of a vertebra which are almost wholly made up of compact bone. This porosity of the cancellous tissue caused by osteoporosis leads to a cavity formation within the affected vertebral body with a partial

TRANSVERSE SECTION OF A VERTEBRA

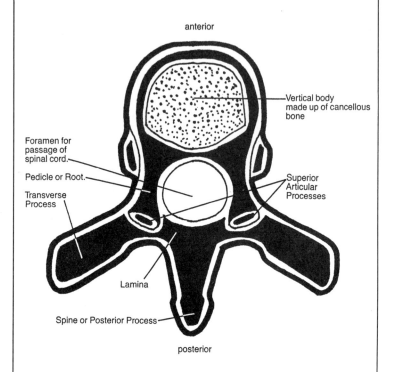

anterior

Vertical body made up of cancellous bone

Foramen for passage of spinal cord.

Pedicle or Root.

Transverse Process

Superior Articular Processes

Lamina

Spine or Posterior Process

posterior

The Vertebral Arch composed of compact bone. It consists of:
(i) a pair of Pedicles, and (ii) 7 Processes, [ie, 4 Articular (facets),
2 Superior only are shown
2 Transverse, or Lateral, and
1 Posterior.]

collapse of this structure. This causes pain and deformity which are the symptoms of the condition.

Before we can appreciate why only the body of the vertebra is affected by this condition, the anatomical and histological make-up of the whole vertebra must be clearly understood.

COMPONENT PARTS OF A VERTEBRA

A vertebra consists of two essential parts, the front or anterior segment called the **body** and the rear or posterior segment which is called the vertebral **arch.** These anterior and posterior processes join to enclose the spinal cord and protect it.

The anterior processes or bodies form a pillar for the support of the head and the trunk, and the column is articulated to allow free movement. The **body** is the largest part of the vertebra, and is more or less cylindrical in shape. The upper and lower surfaces are impaled hyaline cartilaginous plates which have a smooth outer surface against which the disc or nucleus pulposus lies. Around the rim of the body is the strong annular ligament which joins the opposing bodies, encloses the nucleus pulposus and acts as a coil spring to the whole spinal column.

The vertebral **arch** consists of a pair of pedicles or roots. It supports seven processes, four articular processes called facets, two transverse or lateral and one posterior.

The normal vertebra is, as already suggested, made up of two distinct types of bone. The vertebral or neural **arch** and its processes are chiefly composed of **compact bone,** the amount of cancellous tissue being for the most part very small. This strong structure protects the spinal cord and, in not a single case in my experience, was there any evidence of osteoporosis in the compact bone in this area. The vertebral **body** itself, however, is composed of **cancellous tissue,** covered by a thin layer of compact bone.

NUCLEUS EXPANSION OR SCHMORL'S NODES

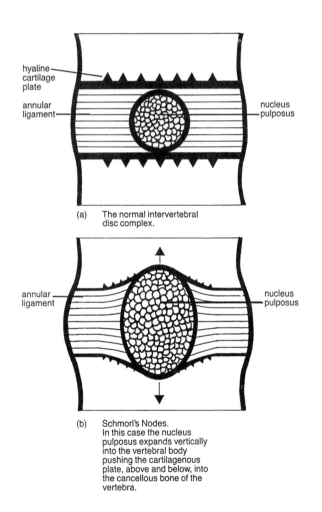

hyaline
cartilage
plate

annular
ligament

nucleus
pulposus

(a) The normal intervertebral
disc complex.

annular
ligament

nucleus
pulposus

(b) Schmorl's Nodes.
In this case the nucleus
pulposus expands vertically
into the vertebral body
pushing the cartilagenous
plate, above and below, into
the cancellous bone of the
vertebra.

204

RESEARCH FINDINGS

During my research into the slipped disc condition which took place in the Pathology Department of the Glasgow Royal Infirmary, it was quite common to come across cases of osteoporosis especially in the older age groups, about 65 years and over. On dissecting the affected segments of the spinal column, I noted that the compact bone enclosing the vertebral body was often practically absent in many areas, and many cases revealed very marked thinning with hair-line fractures of the compact bone. When the thin layer of compact bone covering the vertebral body was stripped off, the underlying cancellous bone showed a sieve-like structure. Also in some cases when the hyaline cartilaginous plates, which are normally impaled into the superior and inferior aspects of the vertebral bodies, were removed, a similar sieve-like state was present on the denuded surface of the vertebral body.

The annual ligaments in some specimens remained intact, but in 50% of the cases the nucleus pulposus or spinal disc had penetrated into the vertebral body and the disc was swollen and enlarged. In many dissections histology revealed no evidence of hyaline cartilage plates. It is, therefore, quite possible that the hyaline cartilage plates were not present at birth or were so extremely thin that they permitted the disc to compress upwards or downwards into the cancellous bone of the vertebral body causing 'nucleus expansion' which is known as **Schmorl's nodes** (see diagram opposite).

CAUSES OF OSTEOPOROSIS

The causes of osteoporosis are not firmly established. It may well be due to an embryological failure. The compact bone around the vertebral body may have failed to become strong enough to perform its function to enclose and protect the vertebral body; or there may have been a failure in the development of the cartilage plates. These causes have been suggested by the evidence of the histological research in the Pathology Department.

Another theory as to its cause is hormonal imbalance particularly during the menopausal cycle, as I have already explained.

However, osteoporosis may also be due to the decalcification of the vertebral body, which may itself be caused by a congenital deficiency of calcium or, in older age groups, to a deficiency of calcium in the diet, or even failure to absorb sufficient calcium by the bowel. This deficiency can be clearly illustrated by an analysis of the patient's blood in the laboratory.

My treatment (see later paragraph) is largely based on this theory and has proved beneficial.

DIAGNOSIS

First, however, correct diagnosis of this condition has to be established and the only sure way of diagnosing it is by X-ray. A lateral radiograph of the spinal column will show positive findings. With the exception of the anterior borders of the bodies, the outlines of the vertebra will be clearly defined; the upper and lower margins of the bodies cast relatively dense linear shadows which may be $1/32''$ thick. Often not the slightest trace of structure may be seen within these bodies, but it is usually just possible to distinguish the anterior surface of the bodies by their slightly greater density. The intervertebral discs are usually swollen and may be half as deep again in the mid-depth of the vertebral bodies. The antero-posterior X-ray will show a decrease in the depth of the affected vertebral bodies. X-rays of the pelvis and limb bones will not usually show any recognisable departure from the normal. There is no evidence of past or present rickets and none of the deformities of osteomalacia, osteogenesis imperfecta or osteitis fibrosa cystica.

The X-ray will also show that in some cases the annular ligament is wholly absent or only partially complete. In these cases, the vertebrae are resting one upon the other with little or no cushioning between them. Often osteophytes, small outgrowths of bone, have grown both upwards and downwards from the vertebral bodies and the pressure exerted on these may cause the vertebrae to become misaligned. In these cases deformity and stiffness of the back will take place, giving rise to varying degrees of pain.

TREATMENT

ANABOLIC STEROIDS

It has been suggested that anabolic steroids have value in reversing bone loss but their major drawbacks, hirsutism and salt and water retention — the latter may result in heart failure particularly in the elderly — make these, to me, at any rate, an unacceptable form of treatment.

HORMONE TREATMENT

As I have already explained, very small weekly doses of oestrogen may be given to female patients of the menopausal age, in addition to my normal prescription of calcium and Vitamin D (see next section). However, where there has been a marked hormonal imbalance I have found that the simple use of calcium and Vitamin D added is in these cases poorly absorbed from the gut. Thus the condition will progress unchecked. In these cases therefore, I prescribe a specialised form of Vitamin D therapy:

one alph 0.25 mic

= 0.25 microgram Affacalcidol

= (α hydrony Vitamin D3)

This has shown to be of value in the fact that the calcium will now be absorbed through the bloodstream into the bones which have a deficiency of calcium.

RECALCIFICATION TREATMENT

Primarily, my treatment aims to recalcify the bones that show evidence of osteoporosis, by prescribing a supplementary daily intake of calcium. Calcium, however, will not be absorbed into the bloodstream without the presence of Vitamin D so that even a diet with a high calcium content will not be absorbed into the system if the calcium is not accompanied by Vitamin D.

In the first phase calcium tablets, with Vitamin D added, are prescribed: two tablets, three times a day. They should be taken in the middle of each meal, so that they are digested and absorbed from the bowel directly into the bloodsteam. Thus any deficient areas of bone i.e. mainly the vertebral bodies, are gradually recalcified. This process of re-ossification may take three to six months to stabilise, and its progress can only be confirmed by X-ray and a lessening of pain in the affected areas.

The second phase, i.e. the correction of deformities caused by osteoporosis is then carried out using gentle surgical manipulation once I am completely satisfied that the condition is under control.

The patient is advised to continue to take a reduced dose of calcium plus Vitamin D, say just one per day with lunch for a further period of six months. Meanwhile the patient reports back to me every three months for a check-up. A sample of blood is taken to check the calcium level in the blood. If this is low the the medication is increased greatly. If pain persists one paracetamol tablet may be taken every four hours but their frequency reduced as pain and discomfort diminish.

The pharmocological make-up of the calcium and Vitamin D tablet that I prescribe is as follows: Calcium Sodium Lactate 450 m.g. Calcium Phosphate 150 m.g. Calciferos 12.5 m.g. equivalent 500 units Vit. D. Activity.

Above all, I counsel my patients to include in their diet, foods which are rich in calcium, for example, dairy produce, milk and cheese; leafy green vegetables, including broccoli and spinach and fish, especially salmon. I also recommend they should take a course of multi vitamin tablets, taking one per day.